Study Guide to Accompany

Focus on Nursing Pharmacology

D0862382

Second Edition

Amy M. Karch, RN, MS
Assistant Professor of Clinical Nursing
University of Rochester School of Nursing
Rochester, New York

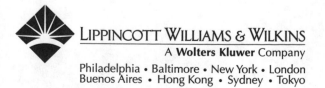

LIPPINCOTT WILLIAMS & WILKINS
A **Wolters Kluwer** Company

Philadelphia • Baltimore • New York • London
Buenos Aires • Hong Kong • Sydney • Tokyo

Acquisitions Editor: Margaret Zuccarini
Managing Editor: Barclay Cunningham
Editorial Assistant: Helen Kogut
Production Editor: Nicole Walz
Senior Production Manager: Helen Ewan
Managing Editor / Production: Erika Kors
Art Director: Carolyn O'Brien
Manufacturing Manager: William Alberti
Compositor: Peirce Graphic Services
Printer: Victor Graphics

2nd Edition

9 8 7 6 5 4 3 2 1

ISBN: 0-7817-3658-7

Introduction

This workbook-style study guide is written to accompany the 2nd edition of *Focus on Nursing Pharmacology*. It is designed to provide practice at word recognition, vocabulary skills, and repeated exposure to the terms, concepts, and application of pharmacology. Having the opportunity to use new vocabulary words and concepts immediately after reading about them in the textbook provides a learning opportunity and a chance to apply the new knowledge in a non-threatening environment. The book consists of a variety of puzzles aimed at repetition and improved learning, and various opportunities to apply the drug information to patient situations. It is hoped that you will be challenged but will also enjoy the review process. Pharmacology can be confusing and sometimes even intimidating, but in this format, it can also be fun. You will find that new words are now familiar terms and that you are comfortable and confident with the new material.

Contents

CHAPTER 1

Introduction to Drugs

■ Matching

Match the word with the appropriate definition.

1. _____ genetic engineering
2. _____ Food and Drug Administration (FDA)
3. _____ pharmacology
4. _____ Phase I study
5. _____ over-the-counter (OTC) drugs
6. _____ preclinical study
7. _____ teratogenic
8. _____ pharmacotherapeutics
9. _____ generic drugs
10. _____ drugs

A. The study of the actions of chemicals on living organisms
B. Drugs sold by their chemical names, not brand-name products
C. Having adverse effects on the fetus
D. Chemicals that are introduced into the body to bring about some sort of change
E. A drug that is available without a prescription
F. Federal agency responsible for the regulation and enforcement of drug evaluation and distribution policies
G. Process of altering deoxyribonucleic acid (DNA) to produce a chemical to be used as a drug
H. Pilot study of a potential drug conducted with a small number of selected, healthy human volunteers
I. Initial trial of a chemical believed to have therapeutic potential; uses laboratory animals, not human subjects
J. Clinical pharmacology, the branch of pharmacology that deals with drugs

■ Web Exercise

Go to the FDA home page on the Internet. Locate the Center for Drug Evaluation and Research (CDER) page. Find one drug that was released within the past 3 months. (The FDA site will list drugs approved by year and month. Click on a year and then a month, and then scroll down the page to find a drug.) Identify the brand name, generic name, and therapeutic class of the drug. Go to the manufacturer's website to get specific information regarding the therapeutic use, adverse effects, and dosage of the drug. (This can be done by entering the generic name of the drug into a search.) Return to the FDA site and try this search for another drug released within the past 3 months.

■ Use of Terms

Identify the correct terms used for the following drugs.

chlordiazepoxide hydrochloride

methaminodiazepoxide hydrochloride

Librium

Pregnancy category B

Benzodiazepine

Antianxiety agent

Therapeutic class

Safety for use during pregnancy

Chemical name

Generic name

Pharmacological class

Brand name

■ Definitions

Write definitions for the following terms.

1. pharmacology _____

_____

2. pharmacotherapeutics _____

_____

3. genetic engineering _____

_____

4. preclinical trials _____

_____

5. generic name _____

_____

6. orphan drug _____

_____

7. OTC drugs _____

_____

8. FDA pregnancy category _____

_____

■ Fill in the Blanks

Describe what occurs in each phase of the drug development process.

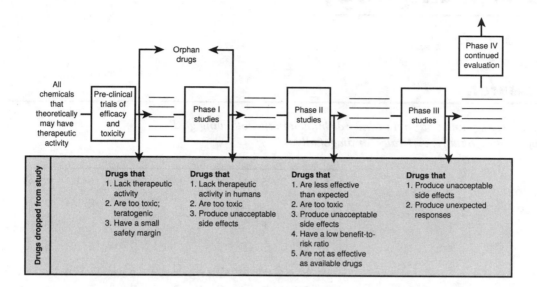

CHAPTER 2

Drugs and the Body

■ Word Search

Circle the following drug- and body-related words hidden in the following grid.
Words may appear horizontally, vertically, or diagonally.

absorption
biotransformation
chemotherapeutic
concentration
critical
distribution
excretion
first-pass
half-life
pharmacodynamics
pharmacokinetics
receptor
site
selective
toxicity

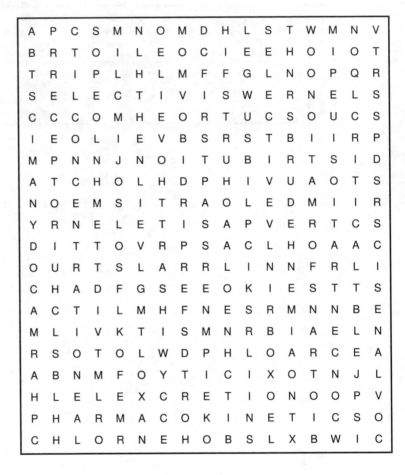

■ Fill in the Blanks

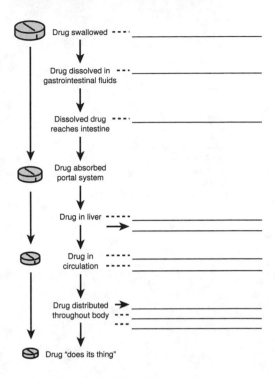

Drug swallowed - - - - _____

Drug dissolved in - - - - _____
gastrointestinal fluids

Dissolved drug - - - - _____
reaches intestine

Drug absorbed
portal system

Drug in liver - - - - - _____
→ _____

Drug in - - - - _____
circulation - - - - _____

Drug distributed → _____
throughout body - - - _____
- - - _____

Drug "does its thing"

■ Multiple Choice

Select the best answer to the following questions.

1. The absorption of a drug given intramuscularly (IM) can be affected by:
   a. food in the stomach.
   b. patient's age.
   c. blood supply to the area injected.
   d. presence of interacting foods in the stomach.

2. The absorption of a drug given subcutaneously (SC) can be affected by:
   a. age of the patient.
   b. temperature of the drug being given.
   c. fat content of the tissue being injected.
   d. muscle tension.

3. The half-life of a drug is 1 hour. A patient receives 50 mg of the drug. The expected concentration in 2 hours would be:
   a. 25 mg.
   b. 12.5 mg.
   c. 10 mg.
   d. 0 mg.

4. Drugs do *not* act at specific receptor sites to:
   a. increase the activity of the cell.
   b. decrease the activity of the cell.
   c. block the receptor site to prevent stimulation.
   d. change the make-up and function of the cell.

5. Excretion of drugs from the body does *not* occur:
   a. from the kidneys.
   b. from the pancreas.
   c. from the lungs.
   d. through the gastrointestinal (GI) tract.

6. The critical concentration of a drug is the amount of a drug:
   a. that will kill a laboratory animal.
   b. that will cause teratogenic effects.
   c. needed to achieve the desired therapeutic effects.
   d. needed in each dose.

7. Distribution involves:
   a. the movement of a drug from the GI tract to the blood stream.
   b. the movement of a drug to the body's tissues.
   c. the breakdown of a drug in the liver.
   d. the removal of a drug from the body at the kidney.

8. Pathological factors do not alter the pharmacokinetics of a drug by affecting:
   a. biotransformation.
   b. excretion.
   c. delivery of the blood to the tissues.
   d. genetic predisposition to adverse effects.

■ Word Scramble

Unscramble the following letters to form words related to pharmacotherapeutics.

1. tsrmafaomrtnioibo _____
2. sittriobnudi _____
3. cobplea _____
4. xncoriete _____
5. msacciotkeinprha _____
6. ptoercer sstie _____
7. llffiahe _____
8. tchietruaepmeoch _____

CHAPTER 3

Toxic Effects of Drugs

■ Definitions

Describe the following adverse reactions.

1. anaphylactic reaction _____

   _____

2. cytotoxic reaction _____

   _____

3. serum sickness reaction _____

   _____

4. superinfection _____

   _____

5. blood dyscrasia _____

   _____

6. hypersensitivity reaction _____

   _____

7. stomatitis _____

   _____

■ Matching

Match the adverse drug effect with the appropriate intervention.

1. _____ hypoglycemia
2. _____ hyperglycemia
3. _____ hypokalemia
4. _____ superinfection
5. _____ cholinergic effects
6. _____ Parkinson-like effects

A. Replace serum potassium and carefully monitor serum levels; provide supportive therapy (safety precautions to prevent injury or falls, orient patient, comfort measures for pain and discomfort).

B. Provide sugarless lozenges, mouth care to help mouth dryness. Arrange for bowel program; have the patient void before taking the drug; provide safety measures if vision changes occur.

C. Administer insulin therapy to decrease blood glucose as appropriate; provide support to help the patient deal with signs and symptoms (access to bathroom facilities, controlled environment, reassurance, mouth care).

D. Discontinue the drug, if necessary; treat with anticholinergics or antiparkinson drugs if recommended and if the benefit outweighs the discomfort of adverse effects; provide small, frequent meals if swallowing becomes difficult; provide safety measures.

E. Restore glucose intravenously (IV) or orally (PO), if possible; provide supportive measures (skin care, environmental control of light and temperature, rest). Institute safety measures to prevent injury or falls.

F. Provide supportive measures (frequent mouth care, skin care, access to bathroom facilities, small and frequent meals); administer antifungal therapy as appropriate.

■ Fill in the Blanks

1. Renal injury is a frequent adverse effect associated with
   _____.

2. Glipizide and glyburide, antidiabetic agents, may cause
   _____, and the patient should be monitored for cool and clammy skin, rapid heart rate, increased blood pressure, and rapid and shallow respirations.

3. Retinal damage and even blindness have been associated with the antirheumatoid agent _____.

4. Dizziness, ringing in the ears, loss of balance, and impaired hearing can occur with aspirin therapy and are referred to as _____.

5. A common adverse effect associated with chemotherapy is
   _____, which can lead to increased bleeding, increased risk of infection, and fatigue.

6. Patients should be advised to avoid driving or operating machinery and other safety precautions should be taken if the patient has central nervous system (CNS) effects such as _____.

CHAPTER 4

Nursing Management

■ Listing

List the seven points to consider in the safe and effective administration of a drug.

1. _____

2. _____

3. _____

4. _____

5. _____

6. _____

7. _____

■ Fill in the Blanks

Fill in the blanks in the following nursing process chart.

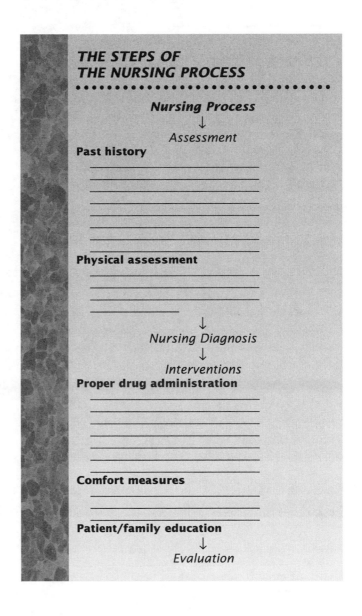

THE STEPS OF
THE NURSING PROCESS
• •

Nursing Process
↓
Assessment

Past history
_____
_____
_____
_____
_____
_____

Physical assessment
_____
_____
_____
_____

↓

Nursing Diagnosis
↓
Interventions

Proper drug administration
_____
_____
_____
_____
_____
_____

Comfort measures
_____
_____
_____

Patient/family education
↓
Evaluation

■ Listing

List eight factors that should always be considered when preparing a patient teaching plan for drug therapy.

1. _____

2. _____

3. _____

4. _____

5. _____

6. _____

7. _____

8. _____

CHAPTER 5

Dosage Calculations

■ Matching

Match the word with the appropriate definition.

1. _____ apothecary system
2. _____ Fried's Rule
3. _____ metric system
4. _____ Young's Rule
5. _____ household system
6. _____ Clark's Rule

A. A method of conversion from adult dose to pediatric dose that assumes that an adult dose would be appropriate for a child who is 12.5 years of age.

B. A method of conversion from adult dose to pediatric dose based on the child's weight.

C. A method of conversion from adult dose to pediatric dose for children 1 to 12 years of age.

D. A system of measure using teaspoons and cups.

E. A system of measure based on the minim and the grain and originally developed for use by pharmacists.

F. A system of measure based on the decimal system and using the gram and liter.

■ Dosage Calculations

Complete the following problems.

1. Change to equivalents within the system:
   a. 100 mg = _____ g
   b. 1500 g = _____ kg
   c. 0.1 L = _____ mL
   d. 500 mL = _____ L

2. Convert to units in the metric system:
   a. 150 gr = _____ g
   b. 1/4 gr = _____ mg
   c. 45 min = _____ mL
   d. 2 qt = _____ L

3. Convert to units in the household system:
   a. 5 mL = _____ tsp
   b. 30 mL = _____ tbs

4. Convert the weights in the following problems:

   a. A patient weighs 170 lb. What is the patient's weight in kilograms?

   170 lb = _____ kg

   b. A patient weighs 3200 g. What is the patient's weight in pounds?

   3200 g = _____ lb

5. Robitussin cough syrup 225 mg PO is ordered. The bottle reads: 600 mg in 1 ounce. How much cough syrup should be given? _____ mL

6. An order is written for *Mellaril* 0.1 g PO q8h. *Mellaril* is available as 30 mg = 1 mL. How much should be given? _____ mL

7. Chloramphenicol is ordered at 0.5 g PO q6h. Available for use are 250-mg chloramphenicol capsules.

   a. How many capsules should be given at each dose? _____ capsules

   b. How many milligrams of chloramphenicol are being given at each dose? _____ mg

8. A postoperative order is written for 1/4 gr codeine q4h as needed (prn) for pain. Each dose given will contain how many milligrams of codeine? _____ mg

9. 240 mg liquid ferrous sulfate is needed for the patient. Available ferrous sulfate contains 40 mg in each mL. How much should be given? _____ mL

10. A patient is given 1 g *Orinase* after breakfast and 0.5 g after lunch. 500-mg *Orinase* tablets are available.

    a. How many tablets are given after breakfast? _____ tablets

    After lunch? _____ tablets

    b. How many milligrams of *Orinase* does the patient receive each day? _____ mg

11. Ordered: 6.5 mg   Available: 10 mg/mL   Proper dose: _____ mL

12. Ordered: 0.35 mg   Available: 1.2 mg/2 mL   Proper dose: _____ mL

13. Ordered: 80 mg   Available: 50 mg/mL   Proper dose: _____ mL

14. Ordered: 150,000 U   Available: 400,000 U/5 mL   Proper dose: _____ mL

15. Ordered: 75,000 U   Available: 500,000 U/10 mL   Proper dose: _____ mL

16. Ordered: 1.5 g   Available: 500 mg/mL   Proper dose: _____ mL

17. Ordered: 1200 mg   Available: 2.5 g/5 mL   Proper dose: _____ mL

18. Ordered: 100 mg   Available: 500 mg/2.5 mL   Proper dose: _____ mL

19. 250 mL of packed cells are to run in over 2 hours. The intravenous (IV) blood set has a drip factor of 6. What should the flow rate be? _____ mL/h; _____ drops/min

20. 500 mL of D5W is to run in over 4 hours. The IV drip factor is 10. What should the flow rate be? _____ mL/h; _____ drops/min

■ Multiple Choice

1. Digoxin 0.25 mg is ordered for a patient who is having trouble swallowing. The bottle of digoxin elixir reads: 0.5 mg/2 mL. How many milliliters would you give?

   a. 50 mL

   b. 0.50 mL

   c. 2.5 mL

   d. 1 mL

2. The usual adult dose of *Benadryl* is 50 mg. What would be the safe dose for a 27-lb child?

   a. 0.9 mg

   b. 1.8 mg

   c. 9.0 mg

   d. 180 mg

3. An order is written for 700 mg ampicillin PO. The drug is supplied in a liquid form as 1 g/3.5 mL. How much of the liquid should be given?

   a. 5.5 mL

   b. 25 mL

   c. 6.25 mL

   d. 2.45 mL

4. An order is written for 1000 mL of normal saline to run in over 10 hours. The drop factor on the IV tubing states 15 drops/mL. What is the IV flow rate?

   a. 50 mL/hr at 50 drops/min

   b. 100 mL/hr at 25 drops/min

   c. 100 mL/hr at 100 drops/min

   d. 50 mL/hr at 15 drop/min

5. The average adult dose of meperidine is 75 mg. What dose would be appropriate for a 10-month-old infant?

   a. 50 mg

   b. 5 mg

   c. 15 mg

   d. 0.5 mg

6. A patient needs to take 0.75 g PO of tetracycline. The drug comes in 250-mg tablets. How many tablets should the patient take?

   a. 12 tablets

   b. 3 tablets

   c. 4 tablets

   d. 13 tablets

7. Aminophylline is supplied in a 500 mg/2.5 mL solution. How much would be given if an order was written for 100 mg aminophylline IV?

    a. 5 mL

    b. 25 mL

    c. 2.5 mL

    d. 0.5 mL

8. 800 U of heparin is ordered for a patient. The heparin is supplied in a multidose vial that is labeled: 10,000 U/mL. How many mL of heparin would be needed to treat this patient?

    a. 0.8 mL

    b. 0.08 mL

    c. 8.0 mL

    d. 0.04 mL

CHAPTER 6

Drug Therapy in the 21st Century

■ Matching

Match the following Internet addresses with the appropriate classification.

1. _____ www.fda.gov
2. _____ www.amhrt.org
3. _____ www.pain.com
4. _____ www.anesthesia.net
5. _____ www.geocities.com
6. _____ www.healthy.net
7. _____ www.healthtouch.com
8. _____ www.nih.gov
9. _____ www.brockport.edu
10. _____ www.monroecc.edu

A. A commercial site that includes advertising, sales, and business
B. An educational site from a school, college, or university
C. A government-sponsored site
D. An official organization site
E. Part of a linked, interconnected network

■ Word Search

Circle the following popular alternative therapies hidden in the following grid.
Words may appear horizontally, vertically, or diagonally.

alfalfa
aloe
bilberry
black cohosh
camomile
chicory
dandelion
echinacea
ephedra
eucalyptus
fenugreek
ginger
ginkobe
ginseng
kava
licorice
rosemary
saw palmetto
tarragon
valerian

A	S	D	A	N	D	E	L	I	O	N	O	B	E	K	J	I	L	M	O	R
B	K	O	L	E	A	N	D	G	I	N	K	O	B	E	L	I	O	N	F	S
O	A	L	O	E	K	A	V	I	L	S	M	R	I	E	P	H	E	D	R	A
S	V	A	L	E	R	I	A	N	P	E	U	C	A	L	Y	P	T	U	S	W
A	A	I	I	P	O	C	H	S	H	C	H	C	H	I	C	O	R	Y	A	P
W	S	L	C	H	S	H	R	E	E	S	I	L	E	M	L	R	I	L	W	A
A	P	I	O	O	E	N	M	N	B	I	O	N	D	O	A	N	D	A	P	L
S	I	L	R	O	M	A	R	G	I	N	G	E	R	M	E	S	L	E	E	M
L	M	S	I	V	A	L	F	A	L	F	A	V	A	A	L	O	I	R	P	E
I	S	L	C	K	R	P	T	D	B	L	A	C	K	C	O	H	O	S	H	T
N	O	M	E	O	Y	O	K	I	E	C	H	I	N	A	C	E	A	H	R	T
G	E	R	C	F	E	N	U	G	R	E	E	K	I	Y	U	Y	U	N	L	O
O	D	O	H	U	R	T	A	R	R	A	G	O	N	H	S	P	L	R	T	N
L	D	S	I	N	G	R	V	E	Y	R	N	M	K	N	L	T	I	L	O	S

■ Definitions

Define the following terms.

1. self-care _____

   _____

2. Internet _____

   _____

3. over-the-counter (OTC) drugs _____

   _____

4. alternative therapies _____

   _____

5. off-label uses _____

   _____

6. cost comparisons _____

   _____

CHAPTER 7

Introduction to Cell Physiology

■ Web Exercise

Look up information on cell physiology, theories of cell formation, and ongoing cellular research at http://www.historyoftheuniverse.com/cell.html. Correlate the structure of the cell membrane with the cell processes discussed in this chapter.

■ Fill in the Blanks

Label the parts of a cell.

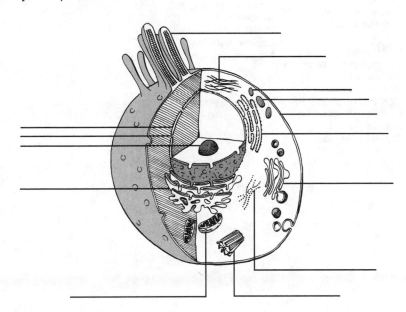

■ Word Scramble

Unscramble the following letters to find basic cellular processes.

1. ifsnofidu _____

2. ctoyseondsi _____

3. ipysonictos _____

4. shipgoytacos _____

5. smooiss _____

6. tosimsi _____

7. vissape tatrrsopn _____

8. evicate protstran _____

■ Matching

Match the phase of the cell cycle with the cell activity during that phase.

1. _____ G$_0$ phase
2. _____ G$_1$ phase
3. _____ S phase
4. _____ G$_2$ phase
5. _____ M phase

A. Cell splits to form two identical daughter cells
B. Synthesis of DNA
C. Manufacture of substances needed to form mitotic spindles
D. Synthesis of substances needed for DNA production
E. Resting phase

■ Crossword Puzzle

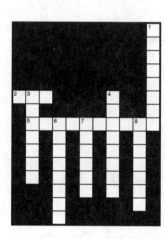

ACROSS

2 Messenger and transcription acids within a cell
5 Part of the genetic make-up of cells

DOWN

1 Lipoprotein substance that protects a cell from its environment
3 Center of a cell containing the genetic material
4 Digestive enzymes found within a cell

6 Site of protein production within a cell
7 Alteration in cell make-up resulting in a different cell membrane or make-up
8 Cell division to form two new daughter cells

CHAPTER 8

Anti-infective Agents

■ Definitions

Define the following terms.

1. culture _____
   _____

2. prophylaxis _____
   _____

3. resistance _____
   _____

4. selective toxicity _____
   _____

5. sensitivity testing _____
   _____

6. spectrum _____
   _____

■ Crossword Puzzle

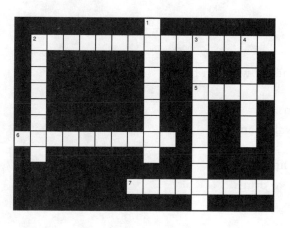

ACROSS

2 Antibiotics that interfere with protein synthesis
5 Basic units of life
6 Antibiotic class developed from molds
7 Ranges of anti-infective activity

DOWN

1 Production of certain substances by a cell

2 Type of immunity that develops after exposure to an organism
3 Ability of a chemical to affect only certain types of cells
4 First scientist to develop a synthetic anti-infective

■ Matching

Match the antibiotic with the appropriate description.

1. _____ polymyxin B

2. _____ meropenem

3. _____ chloramphenicol

4. _____ vancomycin

5. _____ spectinomycin

6. _____ bacitracin

A. Can cause potentially fatal pseudomembranous colitis

B. Associated with "gray-baby" syndrome

C. Very toxic to human cells; nephrotoxicity, neurotoxicity common

D. Its use led to development of many resistant strains

E. Used for staphylococci infections in patients who cannot take penicillin or cephalosporins

F. Treatment of specific strains of *Neisseria gonorrhoeae*

■ Multiple Choice

Select the best answer to the following.

1. Anti-infectives that are being used to prevent infections before they occur are being used for:
   a. sensitivity testing.
   b. broad-spectrum coverage.
   c. prophylaxis.
   d. superinfections.

2. Sensitivity testing is done to:
   a. identify the species of the infecting pathogen.
   b. prevent further illness.
   c. determine the proper dose of the drug needed.
   d. show which drugs are capable of controlling the infecting organism.

3. Microorganisms can develop resistance by:
   a. altering binding sites on the membrane of ribosomes so that they no longer accept the drug.
   b. multiplying less rapidly than usual.
   c. shrinking in on themselves to prevent access to the drug.
   d. completely changing their genetic make-up.

4. Anti-infectives that interfere with the biosynthesis of a bacterial cell wall can be used in humans because:
   a. bacteria do not make cell walls when they are inside humans.
   b. bacteria have a slightly different composition of their cell wall than do humans and will not affect the human cells.
   c. human cells do not biosynthesize their cell walls after fetal life.
   d. bacteria have thick ergot layers, making them impermeable to drugs.

5. Ways that health care providers can help to prevent the emergence of resistant strains would include all of the following *except:*

    a. using high doses of a drug to eradicate the infecting organism.

    b. assuring a long duration of drug use to eradicate the infecting organism.

    c. ordering antibiotics immediately, even if the infecting organism is not known.

    d. using the correct drug, as identified in sensitivity testing to treat the infection.

CHAPTER 9

Antibiotics

■ True or False

Indicate whether the following statements are true (T) or false (F).

_____ 1. Aerobic bacteria depend on oxygen for survival.

_____ 2. Bactericidal refers to a substance that prevents the replication of bacteria.

_____ 3. Bacteriostatic refers to a drug that causes the death of bacteria.

_____ 4. Anaerobic bacteria survive without oxygen.

_____ 5. Gram-negative refers to bacteria that take a positive stain and are frequently associated with infections of the respiratory tract and soft tissues.

_____ 6. An antibiotic is a chemical that inhibits the growth of specific bacteria or causes the death of susceptible bacteria.

_____ 7. Antibiotics usually eradicate all of the bacteria that have entered the body.

_____ 8. Synergistic drugs are drugs that work together to increase a drug's effectiveness.

■ Web Exercise

Go to http://www.cdc.gov. Select Health Topics A-Z, select the letter T, and then find tuberculosis. Develop an information sheet for a patient with tuberculosis, including teaching points, ways to remember to take the medication, family pointers, and drug effects.

■ Word Scramble

Unscramble the following letters to form the names of commonly used cephalosporins.

1. pnrciepiha _____

2. lrcfeoa _____

3. xcifeldaor _____

4. afblroecra _____

5. xciemfetzoi _____

6. nettacoef _____

7. toxinefic _____

8. nozfileca _____

■ Matching

Match the following antibiotics with the correct class.

1. _____ minocycline
2. _____ sulfasalazine
3. _____ capreomycin
4. _____ amikacin
5. _____ cefonicid
6. _____ erythromycin
7. _____ enoxacin
8. _____ clindamycin
9. _____ ampicillin
10. _____ levofloxacin
11. _____ gentamicin
12. _____ dapsone

A. Aminoglycosides
B. Cephalosporins
C. Fluoroquinolones
D. Lincosamides
E. Penicillins
F. Sulfonamides
G. Tetracyclines
H. Leprostatic
I. Antimycobacterials
J. Macrolides

CHAPTER 10

Antiviral Agents

■ Identify the Site of Action

Identify the site of action of the following drugs used to treat HIV/AIDS.

1. reverse transcriptase inhibitors _____

   _____

2. protease inhibitors _____

   _____

3. nucleosides _____

   _____

■ Matching

Match the locally acting antiviral drug with the condition it is typically used to treat.

1. _____ idoxuridine
2. _____ imiquimod
3. _____ fomivirsen
4. _____ penciclovir
5. _____ trifluridine
6. _____ vidarabine

A. Herpes simplex eye infections
B. Herpes simplex eye infections not responsive to idoxuridine
C. Cold sores on the face and lips
D. Genital and perianal warts
E. Cytomegalovirus (CMV) retinitis
F. Herpes simplex keratitis

■ Word Scramble

Unscramble the letters to form the names of drugs used to treat influenza and respiratory viruses, herpes, or CMV.

1. mciacflriv _____
2. vtilreismoa _____
3. cgnavcolir _____
4. tardimainne _____
5. cvaiyrocl _____
6. cyvalclaoriv _____
7. timedanana _____

  8. iiirrnvab _____

  9. cronefast _____

 10. inmazariv _____

 11. rviavloglacnic _____

 12. dorcifovi _____

■ Patient Teaching Checklist

Mr. Jones, a 48-year-old piano tuner with a positive HIV titer, has recently begun developing signs of AIDS. He is still asymptomatic but was recently started on zidovudine, 100 mg every 4 hours (q4h) when awake. He has been referred to the nurse for drug teaching. Use the patient teaching checklist format to prepare a drug sheet specifically for Mr. Jones.

■ Fill in the Blanks

 1. A *Diskhaler* is used to deliver _____ to treat uncomplicated influenza A infections in adults and children.

 2. Children with respiratory syncytial virus (RSV) often respond very well to treatment with _____.

 3. Patients with Parkinson's disease who were treated with _____ were found to have a decreased incidence of influenza. This drug is now used to treat and prevent influenza infections.

 4. _____ is only available in intravenous (IV) form and is very renal toxic. It is effective in treating CMV retinitis in immune compromised patients and mucocutaneous acyclovir-resistant herpes simplex infections.

 5. Herpes zoster and recurrent genital herpes are often treated with the oral agent _____.

 6. A very commonly used drug for the treatment of herpes infections is _____ (*Zovirax*).

 7. One of the first drugs approved for treating HIV infections that is still used frequently in combination therapy today is _____, known only as AZT in many communities.

 8. A topical drug that is applied locally for the treatment of cold sores is _____.

CHAPTER 11

Antifungal Agents

■ Web Exercise

The basketball coach at the local high school is concerned about an epidemic of athlete's foot that is affecting his entire team. Go on to the Internet to find information that will allow you to prepare a teaching protocol to help the coach with the treatment and prevention of this problem. Go to http://www.athletesfoot.com/ to get all types of information to help you prepare the teaching protocol; http://www.cdc.gov will give you information about available treatments and preventive measures that should be taken.

■ Word Search

Circle the following names of antifungal drugs hidden in the following grid. Words may appear horizontally, vertically, or diagonally.

amphotericin B
butenafine
butoconazole
clotrimazole
econazole
fluconazole
flucytosine
gentian
violet
itraconazole
ketoconazole
miconazole
naftifine
nystatin
oxiconazole
terbinafine
tolnaftate

T	E	R	B	I	N	A	F	I	N	E	Z	O	L	E	C	O	N	C	T
F	N	O	Z	L	E	T	O	L	N	A	F	T	A	T	E	X	F	O	O
L	I	M	G	R	A	O	L	I	C	B	L	B	C	O	N	K	E	N	H
U	S	F	E	A	N	V	F	J	T	H	E	U	A	N	P	E	L	A	P
C	O	L	T	C	I	I	R	L	U	R	Z	T	R	I	E	T	O	Z	M
O	T	U	U	O	T	O	E	E	N	E	A	O	G	L	R	O	Z	O	A
Z	Y	C	B	F	A	L	L	L	L	N	A	C	B	A	I	C	A	L	C
O	C	O	A	N	T	E	O	O	O	I	C	O	O	R	Z	O	M	E	E
L	U	N	E	A	S	T	Z	Z	Z	F	I	N	N	N	O	N	I	M	B
E	L	A	L	Z	Y	A	A	A	O	A	T	A	F	G	A	A	R	H	U
Y	F	Z	O	L	N	G	N	N	L	N	A	Z	I	E	L	Z	T	L	F
I	R	O	Z	O	E	E	O	O	E	E	N	O	C	N	E	O	O	F	L
N	I	L	C	R	L	N	C	C	V	T	O	L	O	T	S	L	L	L	O
E	N	E	I	O	Z	T	I	I	I	U	L	E	L	I	A	E	C	S	E
B	U	T	O	C	O	I	X	M	O	B	C	R	E	A	B	L	H	T	H
R	L	G	A	M	P	H	O	T	E	R	I	C	I	N	B	E	L	R	A

■ Fill in the Blanks

1. A fungus is a cellular organism with a _____ cell wall that contains chitin and polysaccharides and a cell membrane that contains _____.

2. Any infection with a fungus is called a(n) _____.

3. Systemic antifungals can be very toxic; adverse effects may include _____ and _____ failure.

4. Vaginal and oral yeast infections are often caused by _____.

5. Athlete's foot and jock itch are examples of _____ infections.

6. Topical antifungals can be toxic and should not be absorbed _____.

7. Topical antifungals should not be used near _____ or lesions, which could increase absorption.

8. Topical antifungals can cause serious local _____, _____, and _____.

■ Matching

Match the antifungal with the disorder it is usually used to treat.

1. _____ clotrimazole

2. _____ tolnaftate

3. _____ miconazole

4. _____ econazole

5. _____ haloprogin

6. _____ terbinafine

7. _____ undecylenic acid

8. _____ butoconazole

A. Oral and vaginal mycoses

B. Oral and vaginal *Candida* infections

C. Athlete's foot

D. Tinea infections

E. Vaginal *Candida* infections

F. Topical mycosis

G. Diaper rash, jock itch

H. Jock itch and ringworm

CHAPTER 12

Antiprotozoal Agents

■ Matching

Match the route or causative organism with the associated disease.

1. _____ leishmaniasis
2. _____ amebiasis
3. _____ malaria
4. _____ giardiasis
5. _____ PCP
6. _____ trichomoniasis
7. _____ trypanosomiasis

A. *Pneumocystis carinii*
B. Plasmodium
C. Tsetse fly bite
D. Sand fly bite
E. *Entamoeba histolytica*
F. Intestinal protozoan
G. Vaginal protozoan

■ Fill in the Blanks

Fill in the stages of the life cycle of the Anopheles mosquito.

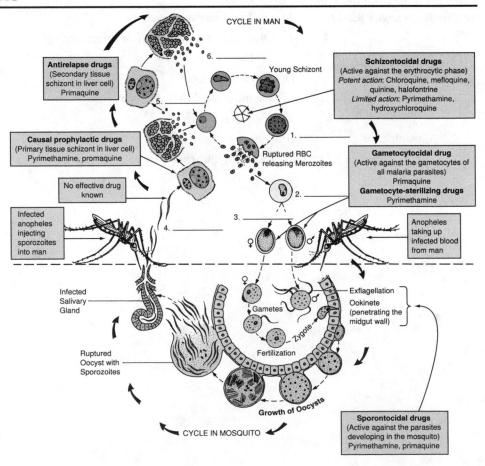

■ Web Exercise

A friend of yours has won a trip around the world to many exotic places.
You are asked if any immunizations are needed before the trip. Go to
http://www.cdc.gov/travel and prepare a summary of suggested vaccinations
or prophylactic measures that should be taken.

■ Matching

Match the following antiprotozoal drugs with the protozoal infection they are used
to treat.

1. _____ primaquine

2. _____ atovaquone

3. _____ quinine

4. _____ pentamidine

5. _____ chloroquine

6. _____ halofantrine

7. _____ metronidazole

8. _____ hydroxychloroquine

A. Malaria

B. PCP infection

C. Trypanosomiasis and leishmaniasis

D. Trichomoniasis, giardiasis, amebiasis

CHAPTER 13

Anthelmintic Agents

■ Definitions

Define the following terms.

1. cestode _____

_____

2. nematode _____

_____

3. pinworm _____

_____

4. roundworm _____

_____

5. schistosomiasis _____

_____

6. trichinosis _____

_____

7. threadworm _____

_____

8. whipworm _____

_____

■ Patient Teaching Checklist

Prepare a patient teaching checklist for an individual who has been diagnosed with pinworms and has been prescribed mebendazole. The patient will be at home during treatment of this disease.

■ Fill in the Blanks

Fill in the phases of the life cycle of the worms associated with schistosomiasis.

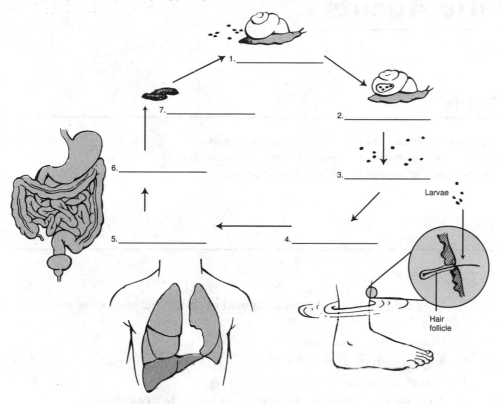

1. _____
2. _____
3. _____
4. _____
5. _____
6. _____
7. _____

Larvae

Hair
follicle

■ Word Search

Circle the following words related to anthelmintic therapy hidden in the following grid. Words may appear horizontally, vertically, or diagonally.

albendazole
cestode
filariasis
helminth
ivermectin
nematode
pinworm
platyhelminth
praziquantel
pyrantel
roundworm
schistosomiasis
thiabendazole
trichinosis
whipworm

T	A	P	E	W	O	R	M	C	E	S	M	E	T	O	D	E	S
S	B	F	H	L	Q	U	A	R	I	R	S	I	S	O	S	I	S
P	A	L	B	E	N	D	A	Z	O	L	E	W	O	R	M	S	E
E	C	I	R	O	U	N	D	W	O	R	M	P	I	N	P	S	E
O	F	F	W	O	R	M	P	Y	R	A	N	T	E	L	I	P	H
L	I	P	S	O	P	I	N	W	O	R	M	H	I	S	N	R	P
W	L	O	I	R	H	M	Q	U	O	S	N	I	A	S	W	A	T
V	A	L	S	W	O	R	M	C	U	T	E	I	L	W	O	Z	M
O	R	M	O	H	E	M	E	E	P	S	M	O	L	T	R	I	U
Q	I	O	N	T	P	I	N	S	S	O	A	S	I	S	M	Q	U
U	A	L	I	N	H	O	R	T	S	M	T	W	L	O	V	U	P
P	S	O	H	I	L	M	T	O	W	O	O	R	M	V	E	A	L
M	I	S	C	M	I	N	T	D	I	L	D	W	O	R	M	N	O
O	S	S	I	L	O	S	S	E	P	I	E	H	E	L	M	T	N
V	O	L	R	E	I	V	E	R	M	E	C	T	I	N	S	E	N
M	E	T	T	H	I	A	B	E	N	D	A	Z	O	L	E	L	O
O	S	O	C	H	T	N	I	M	L	E	H	Y	T	A	L	P	I
L	I	S	O	Q	U	I	A	W	O	R	M	C	A	R	T	S	Q

CHAPTER 14

Antineoplastic Agents

■ Nursing Care Guide

*Jim Jackson has chronic myelogenous leukemia, Philadelphia chromosome positive.
He is scheduled to receive busulfan at the chemotherapy center. Prepare a nursing care
guide for Mr. Jackson to ensure continuity of care during his treatment program.*

■ Matching

Match the word with the appropriate definition.

1. _____ anaplasia
2. _____ alopecia
3. _____ carcinoma
4. _____ metastasize
5. _____ neoplasm
6. _____ sarcoma
7. _____ autonomy
8. _____ antineoplastic

A. Tumors in the mesenchyma, composed of embryonic connective tissue cells
B. Drugs used to combat cancer
C. Tumors starting in epithelial cells
D. Loss of organization and structure
E. To travel throughout the body via lymph and circulation
F. New growth or cancer
G. Loss of hair
H. Loss of normal controls and reactions that limit cell growth and spreading

■ Word Scramble

*Unscramble the following words to form the names of commonly used antineoplastic
agents.*

1. tlvniinsaeb _____
2. mcenualtirs _____
3. cnbporatali _____
4. psnitilac _____
5. fnxiometa _____
6. cmbyloeni _____
7. ezabacadri _____
8. pdeteosoi _____

■ Fill in the Blanks

Identify the phases of the cell cycle that are affected by the types of antineoplastic drugs noted in the following diagram.

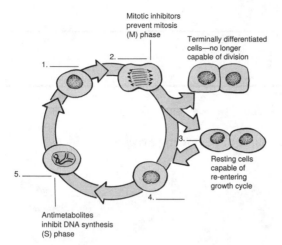

■ Crossword Puzzle

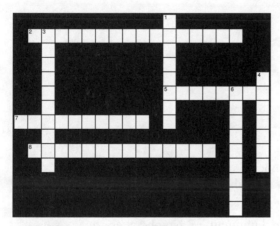

ACROSS

2 Having the ability to protect the heart

5 Loss of hair

7 The ability to enter the lymphatic or circulatory system and move to other parts of the body from the site of origin

8 Having similar characteristics to essential natural substances that are needed for growth and cell division

DOWN

1 A new or cancerous growth

3 Affecting the DNA, RNA, or other cellular proteins and causing cytoxicity

4 A tumor originating in the mesenchyma

6 A tumor originating in the epithelial cells

CHAPTER 15

Introduction to the Immune Response and Inflammation

■ Multiple Choice

Select the best answer to the following.

1. The inflammatory response is characterized by all of the following *except:*
   a. local tissue swelling.
   b. tissue tenderness.
   c. tissue redness.
   d. red blood cell (RBC) phagocytosis.

2. B and T cells are similar in that they both:
   a. secrete antibodies.
   b. play roles in the humoral immune response.
   c. stem from precursors in the bone marrow.
   d. are phagocytic lymphocytes.

3. Antibodies are:
   a. proteins.
   b. secreted by T cells.
   c. enzymes.
   d. effective against any antigens.

4. Specific immune responses involve a B lymphocyte system and a T lymphocyte system. Which of the following statements is true about these systems?
   a. T and B lymphocytes have entered the thymus.
   b. T lymphocytes are involved in cell-mediated immunity; B lymphocytes are involved in antibody-related immunity.
   c. T lymphocytes cannot influence B lymphocyte activity.
   d. T lymphocytes are important in regulating antibody production.

5. Interleukin 2:
   a. is released from leukocytes as a means of communicating with other leukocytes.
   b. causes a decrease in temperature by directly affecting the hypothalamus.
   c. can induce rapid eye movement (REM) sleep stage.
   d. stimulates the production of more B cells in the bone marrow.

6. Clonal theory states that:
   a. each clone of B cells can recognize and bind with many different foreign proteins.

b. humans develop their B clones sometime after birth.

c. plasma cells derive from one clone of B cells and will secrete only one kind of antibody.

d. most humans will be able to develop new B clones when exposed to previously unencountered antigens.

■ Fill in the Blanks

Fill in the following blanks, indicating the clinical signs and symptoms of the inflammatory response and the major catalysts of these signs and symptoms.

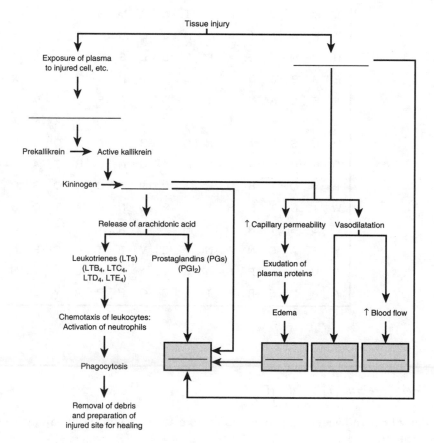

■ Word Search

Circle the following words relating to the immune system and the inflammatory response hidden in the following grid. Words may appear horizontally, vertically, or diagonally.

antibody
arachidonic acid
autoimmune
basophil
chemotaxis
complement
cytotoxin
eosinophil
Hageman factor
interferon
interleukin
kinin
leukocyte
lymphocyte
neutrophil
phagocyte
plasma cell
thymus

B	Q	E	S	T	U	N	L	O	I	P	M	W	R	Y	O	I
D	L	S	H	I	M	N	T	P	S	H	O	H	E	S	C	N
A	C	O	M	P	L	E	M	E	N	T	R	E	S	E	H	T
L	H	S	P	O	I	U	N	R	O	H	E	R	T	R	E	E
H	A	M	F	A	C	T	O	R	R	Y	L	E	I	S	M	R
L	M	R	S	L	B	R	T	A	S	M	B	P	K	X	O	L
K	E	U	A	I	R	O	H	L	E	U	K	O	C	Y	T	E
U	R	M	L	C	A	P	E	S	L	S	E	L	H	N	A	U
E	S	B	E	O	H	H	L	I	O	H	K	Q	N	Y	X	K
L	E	L	A	N	T	I	B	O	D	Y	P	U	I	M	I	I
E	N	Y	M	T	I	L	D	P	E	K	H	I	X	N	S	N
U	U	S	P	I	A	B	O	O	R	I	A	S	O	B	I	K
O	M	P	H	A	G	E	M	A	N	N	G	H	T	A	T	E
L	M	O	I	R	U	R	I	L	O	I	O	E	O	S	R	U
W	I	N	T	E	R	F	E	R	O	N	C	A	T	O	N	E
E	O	S	I	N	O	P	H	I	L	A	Y	A	Y	P	S	O
S	T	A	G	N	A	N	Y	S	V	E	T	E	C	H	N	O
P	U	L	L	P	L	A	S	M	A	C	E	L	L	I	N	K
A	A	P	E	P	E	T	Y	C	O	H	P	M	Y	L	D	Y

■ True or False

Indicate whether the following statements are true (T) or false (F).

_____ 1. You are walking in a daisy field and get stung by what looks like a wasp. You should apply ice to the area to contain the venom.

_____ 2. You have a hard, reddened, warm area on your arm. You should apply ice to the affected area to keep the hardness, redness, and warmth from spreading.

_____ 3. You have a hard, reddened, warm area on your arm. You should apply heat to the area to increase the blood flow to provide inflammatory and immune factors to the site.

_____ 4. Having your tonsils removed will prevent further upper respiratory infections.

_____ 5. Basophils are the first white blood cells at the site of an injury.

_____ 6. All white blood cells possess the property of phagocytosis.

_____ 7. Chemotaxis is the ability to move within the tissues.

_____ 8. Plasma cells are large and active B cells.

_____ 9. The thymus gland is responsible for the activation and programming of the B cells.

_____ 10. Applying ice to an injection site will decrease the pain of the injection but will also decrease the absorption of the injected substance.

CHAPTER 16

Anti-inflammatory Agents

■ Web Exercise

You are caring for a patient who is newly diagnosed with rheumatoid arthritis. The family is involved and supportive and would like information on the disease and treatment options and any new information. Go to http://www.arthritis.org and prepare an information sheet for this family using data from that site.

■ Word Scramble

Unscramble the following letters to form the names of commonly used anti-inflammatory agents.

1. exonrhap _____
2. clausind _____
3. ralooctek _____
4. fidoneccal _____
5. broupfine _____
6. zolasnalie _____
7. thannapoceine _____
8. slataslae _____
9. prisain _____
10. frotnokeep _____

■ Matching

Match the word with the appropriate definition.

1. _____ anti-inflammatory
2. _____ antipyretic
3. _____ analgesic
4. _____ salicylates
5. _____ NSAIDs
6. _____ pyrogens
7. _____ chrysotherapy

A. Treatment with gold salts
B. Nonsteroidal anti-inflammatory drugs
C. Block the prostaglandin system to prevent inflammation
D. Blocking the effects of the inflammatory response
E. Blocking pain sensation
F. Substances that elevate the body's temperature
G. Blocking fever

■ Definitions

Define the following terms.

1. analgesic _____

_____

2. anti-inflammatory _____

_____

3. antipyretic _____

_____

4. chrysotherapy _____

_____

5. NSAIDs _____

_____

6. salicylates _____

_____

7. arthritis _____

_____

8. fever _____

_____

CHAPTER 17

Immune Modulators

■ Definitions

Define the following terms.

1. autoimmune _____

   _____

2. interferon _____

   _____

3. interleukin _____

   _____

4. monoclonal antibodies _____

   _____

5. immune suppressant _____

   _____

■ Matching

Match the interferon with its usual indication for use.

1. _____ interferon alfa-2a

2. _____ interferon alfa-2b

3. _____ interferon alfacon-1-1

4. _____ interferon alfa-n3

5. _____ interferon beta-1a

6. _____ interferon beta-1b

7. _____ interferon gamma-1b

A. Treatment of multiple sclerosis

B. Treatment of leukemias, Kaposi's sarcoma, warts, hepatitis B, malignant melanoma

C. Treatment of multiple sclerosis

D. Treatment of serious, chronic granulomatous disease

E. Treatment of leukemias, Kaposi's sarcoma

F. Treatment of chronic hepatitis C

G. Intralesional treatment of warts

■ Fill in the Blanks

1. _____ _____ are specific antibodies produced by a single clone of B cells to react with a specific antigen.

2. The following monoclonal antibodies are used in the prevention of renal transplant rejection: _____, _____, and _____.

3. Infliximab is used to treat _____ disease in patients who do not respond to other therapy.

4. Palivizumab was developed for the prevention of _____ _____ _____ in children who are at high-risk.

5. Treatment of metastatic breast cancer with tumors that overexpress human epidermal growth factor receptor 2 (HER2) is specifically the indication for _____.

6. _____ is used for the treatment of relapsed follicular B-cell non-Hodgkin's lymphoma B lymphocytes.

7. The treatment of asthma with a strong allergic component is the main indication for _____.

8. _____ is specifically used to treat B cell chronic lymphocytic leukemia.

■ Word Search

Find the names of the following drugs used to affect the immune system hidden in the following grid. The words may appear diagonally, vertically, or horizontally.

aldesleukin
alemtuzumab
azathioprine
basiliximab
cyclosporine
daclizumab
glatiramer
interferon
levamisole
muromonab
mycophenolate
oprelvekin
rituximab
sirolimus
tacrolimus

```
A E T A L O N E H P O C Y M O R A I E D
B N B A M I X I L I S A B A L I Z O P A
O I O A L E M T U Z U M A B A T Z U O C
D R N O Z M A B U Z U M E X O U D A M L
I O I R E A B S L M O L N T U X I B U I
E P K E P M T C O I O L Z U M I C D R Z
A S U M T A R H E S I R O L I M U S O U
N O E A S E L I I O T B R O W A N I M M
T L L R G E O M R O G I A B R B O W O A
I C S I R E A T S O P R E L V E K I N B
L Y E T C V O T T O N R E A R T H I A S
Y C D A E A T A C R O L I M U S S A B G
M O L L I N T E R F E R O N B E A G L E
P E A G L B E V A M I S O L E W E B E R
H O M E P G E A O M A C C O N N E C T I
```

CHAPTER 18

Vaccines and Sera

■ Web Exercise

Your patient, a new mother, has arrived at the clinic with her 2-week-old baby for routine postpartum health care. She has been watching a television talk show about the hazards of vaccinations and asks some good questions about vaccinating her baby. Go to the Internet and find some useful information that can be printed out to help your patient understand vaccinations and to make good decisions about her child's health care.

■ True or False

Indicate whether the following statements are true (T) or false (F).

_____ 1. Tetanus vaccines will provide active immunity against tetanus toxins.

_____ 2. Active immunity occurs when the host is stimulated to make antibodies to a specific antigen.

_____ 3. Gamma globulin provides a good form of passive immunity to patients exposed to a specific antigen.

_____ 4. Vaccines are used to promote active immunity.

_____ 5. Vaccines are only used to prevent infection with future exposures.

_____ 6. Serious reactions have occurred to routine immunizations in the past.

_____ 7. Patients will not experience any discomfort after an immunization injection.

_____ 8. Serum sickness—a massive immune reaction—occurs more frequently with vaccines than with immune sera.

■ Fill in the Blanks

Fill in the blanks in the following figure to indicate the timing of routine immunizations.

Vaccine	Birth	2 mo	4 mo	6 mo	12 mo	15 mo	18 mo	24 mo	4–6 y	11–12 y	14–16 y
Hepatitis B											
Hepatitis B*											
DPT											
Tetanus booster											
H. influenzae b											
Poliovirus (IPV)											
Measles, mumps, rubella											
Varicella											
Hepatitis A†											

*Infants born to HBsAg-positive mothers.
†Recommended in selected areas only, check with your local Health Department.
Suggested by the American Academy of Pediatrics, January, 2000

■ Crossword Puzzle

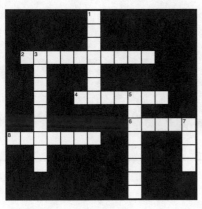

ACROSS

2 Childhood disease with characteristic lesions and scars
4 Agent to stimulate immunity
6 Viral disease
8 Bacterial disease associated with locked jaw presentation

DOWN

1 German measles
3 Inflammation of the liver
5 Resistance to infection
7 Antitoxin

Introduction to Nerves and the Nervous System

■ Fill in the Blanks

Insert the following labels as they apply to the nerve: soma, cell nucleus, dendrites, axon hillock, axon, Schwann cells, and nodes of Ranvier.

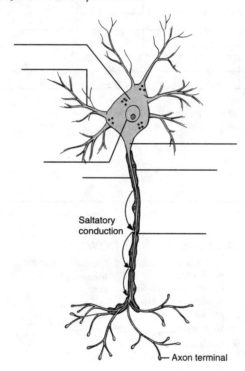

Saltatory conduction

Axon terminal

■ Matching

Match the word with the appropriate definition.

1. _____ action potential
2. _____ afferent
3. _____ axon
4. _____ dendrite
5. _____ depolarization
6. _____ effector
7. _____ efferent
8. _____ engram
9. _____ forebrain
10. _____ hindbrain

A. Motor neurons
B. Long projection from a neuron that carries information from one nerve to another nerve or effector
C. Neurons or groups of neurons that bring information to the CNS
D. The brainstem
E. Upper level of the brain
F. Short-term memory
G. The electrical signal by which neurons send information
H. Muscle, a gland, or another nerve stimulated by a nerve
I. Reversing the membrane charge from negative to positive
J. Short projection on a neuron that transmits information

■ Diagram

Diagram an action potential and label the cellular events that occur during each phase of the action potential.

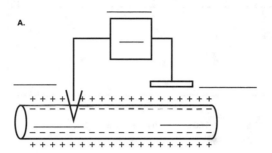

A.

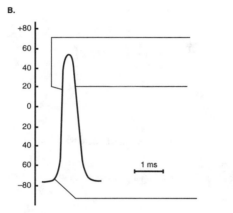

B.

■ Word Search

Circle the following words related to the nervous system hidden in the following grid. Words may appear horizontally, vertically, or diagonally.

action potential
afferent
axon
dendrite
depolarization
effector
efferent
engram
forebrain
hindbrain
limbic system
midbrain
neuron
neurotransmitter
repolarization
Schwann cell
soma
synapse

C	O	N	E	B	U	Y	O	R	E	N	E	R	T	I	A	S	M	A	R	E
O	N	I	P	N	T	J	T	F	D	E	R	E	S	P	A	N	Y	S	N	G
L	O	L	A	I	T	N	E	T	O	P	N	O	I	T	C	A	K	O	E	I
U	F	P	H	A	L	I	M	B	I	C	S	Y	S	T	E	M	I	M	U	E
M	S	E	R	R	Y	Y	I	R	A	V	V	T	N	U	M	T	E	A	R	A
N	C	R	I	B	R	H	J	T	N	E	R	E	F	F	A	L	R	O	O	S
A	H	O	N	E	I	T	A	E	M	E	E	F	O	Z	U	N	I	R	T	K
R	W	N	E	R	C	N	I	A	R	B	D	N	I	H	S	O	N	A	R	I
B	A	E	A	O	A	O	N	D	E	N	D	R	I	T	E	S	S	H	A	N
A	N	T	C	F	C	R	E	P	O	L	A	R	I	Z	A	T	I	O	N	A
N	N	I	E	O	I	M	L	D	Y	L	S	A	O	B	T	M	T	S	S	S
X	C	I	A	X	O	N	L	I	O	T	H	Y	N	O	A	I	N	E	M	I
Y	E	R	T	R	D	I	E	P	A	S	O	A	I	R	G	R	E	N	I	T
P	L	D	Y	I	B	N	E	U	R	O	N	D	G	G	O	R	R	A	T	E
S	L	X	L	M	C	D	K	C	L	N	W	N	D	O	A	O	E	R	T	A
T	S	A	C	A	O	T	I	N	F	Y	E	R	O	T	C	E	F	F	E	P
I	Y	E	O	B	R	K	A	M	R	B	E	U	N	T	N	M	F	F	R	A
L	N	S	L	A	I	R	T	Y	E	O	R	T	T	N	Y	Y	E	O	R	S
P	A	P	I	G	M	A	H	R	D	R	S	A	W	A	W	A	E	R	Y	N

CHAPTER 20

Anxiolytic and Hypnotic Agents

■ Fill in the Blanks

1. _____ is a feeling of tension, nervousness, apprehension, or fear that usually involves unpleasant reactions to a stimulus, which is actual or unknown.

2. Mild anxiety may serve as a stimulus or _____ in some situations.

3. _____ are drugs that can calm patients and make them unaware of their environment.

4. Drugs that can cause sleep are called _____.

5. Anxiolytics can prevent feelings of _____ or _____.

6. Patients who are restless, nervous, irritable, or overreacting to stimuli could benefit from _____.

7. Hypnosis or sleep can be caused by drugs that _____ the central nervous system (CNS).

8. _____ are the most frequently used anxiolytic drugs.

■ Matching

Match the generic name of these commonly used anxiolytic drugs with the associated brand name.

1. _____ clonazepam
2. _____ lorazepam
3. _____ temazepam
4. _____ alprazolam
5. _____ oxazepam
6. _____ triazolam
7. _____ diazepam
8. _____ chlordiazepoxide
9. _____ flurazepam
10. _____ clorazepate

A. *Restoril*
B. *Xanax*
C. *Klonopin*
D. *Valium*
E. *Ativan*
F. *Librium*
G. *Serax*
H. *Halcion*
I. *Tranxene*
J. *Dalmane*

■ Web Exercise

One of your patients has acute anxiety disorder. His family members are upset and feel alone and hopeless. Search the Internet to find support groups and educational information that might help this family.

■ Word Scramble

Unscramble the following letters to form words related to anxiolytic agents.

1. dozzainebipene _____
2. notycpih _____
3. datevise _____
4. ttbbaarriue _____
5. pbiursoen _____
6. pleanolz _____
7. doezmlip _____
8. pezmadia _____
9. tarbblianopeh _____
10. loxtiicayn _____

CHAPTER 21

Antidepressant Agents

■ Multiple Choice

Select the best answer to the following.

1. Affect refers to:
   a. people's feelings in response to their environment.
   b. people's thought processes.
   c. something that is not a normal part of everyday life.
   d. alterations in perceiving the environment

2. Depression:
   a. is always traceable to a precipitating event.
   b. is a common affective disorder.
   c. involves anger and excited states.
   d. is easily diagnosed with the proper tests.

3. Antidepressants may be classified as:
   a. γ-aminobutyric acid (GABA) inhibitors, tricyclics, and selective serotonin reuptake inhibitors (SSRIs).
   b. tricyclic antidepressants (TCAs), the monoamine oxidase (MAO) inhibitors, and the SSRIs.
   c. benzodiazepines, MAO inhibitors, and phenothiazines.
   d. barbiturates, phenothiazines, and miscellaneous drugs.

4. Tricyclic antidepressants:
   a. reduce the release of 5HT and norepinephrine from nerves.
   b. block the metabolism of released 5HT and norepinephrine.
   c. reduce the reuptake of 5HT and norepinephrine by nerves.
   d. occupy specific 5HT and norepinephrine sites on stimulated nerves.

5. Tyramine-containing foods must be limited with the use of MAO inhibitors. Tyramine is found in:
   a. green, leafy vegetables.
   b. yellow fruits and vegetables.
   c. aged cheeses and wines.
   d. chicken—especially white meat.

■ Word Search

Circle the names of the following antidepressants hidden in the following grid. Words may appear horizontally, vertically, or diagonally.

amoxapine
bupropion
citalopram
clomipramine
desipramine
doxepin
imipramine
isocarboxazid
maprotiline
nefazodone
nortriptyline
paroxetine
phenelzine
sertraline
trazodone
venlafaxine

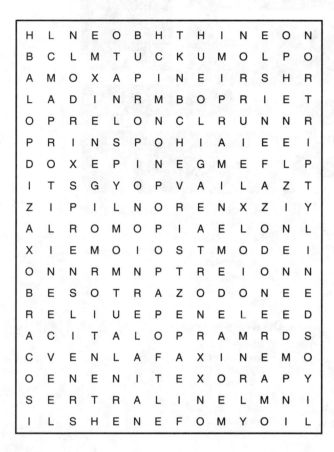

H	L	N	E	O	B	H	T	H	I	N	E	O	N
B	C	L	M	T	U	C	K	U	M	O	L	P	O
A	M	O	X	A	P	I	N	E	I	R	S	H	R
L	A	D	I	N	R	M	B	O	P	R	I	E	T
O	P	R	E	L	O	N	C	L	R	U	N	N	R
P	R	I	N	S	P	O	H	I	A	I	E	E	I
D	O	X	E	P	I	N	E	G	M	E	F	L	P
I	T	S	G	Y	O	P	V	A	I	L	A	Z	T
Z	I	P	I	L	N	O	R	E	N	X	Z	I	Y
A	L	R	O	M	O	P	I	A	E	L	O	N	L
X	I	E	M	O	I	O	S	T	M	O	D	E	I
O	N	N	R	M	N	P	T	R	E	I	O	N	N
B	E	S	O	T	R	A	Z	O	D	O	N	E	E
R	E	L	I	U	E	P	E	N	E	L	E	E	D
A	C	I	T	A	L	O	P	R	A	M	R	D	S
C	V	E	N	L	A	F	A	X	I	N	E	M	O
O	E	N	E	N	I	T	E	X	O	R	A	P	Y
S	E	R	T	R	A	L	I	N	E	L	M	N	I
I	L	S	H	E	N	E	F	O	M	Y	O	I	L

■ Word Scramble

Unscramble the following letters to form the names of commonly used antidepressants.

1. porbpnuio _____

2. otlinuexfe _____

3. mamicoprline _____

4. flaxivenaen _____

5. zipneehlne _____

6. tnexopraei _____

7. pimiminrae _____

8. dozenfaeno _____

■ Crossword Puzzle

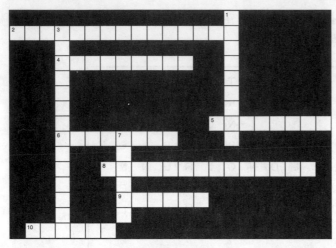

ACROSS

2 Enzyme that breaks down norepinephrine
4 Drug that blocks the reuptake of norepinephrine and serotonin
5 An amine associated with brain chemistry
6 Specific site on a cell that reacts with neurotransmitters
8 Neurotransmitter whose lack is associated with depression
9 State of feeling about one's environment
10 Reabsorption of a chemical into a cell

DOWN

1 Neurotransmitter whose low levels are associated with depression
3 Drug used to relieve affective disorder
associated with sadness and lethargy
7 Popular SSRI

■ Fill in the Blanks

1. The biogenic amines linked to depression include _____, _____, and _____.

2. The MAO inhibitors block the _____ of norepinephrine, leading to an accumulation of that neurotransmitter in the _____.

3. The SSRIs block the _____ of serotonin, leading to an increase in that neurotransmitter near the receptor sites.

4. The tricyclic antidepressants are believed to reduce the reuptake of _____ and _____ in all nerves that produce those neurotransmitters.

5. Because of a risk of increased blood pressure, patients taking MAO inhibitors should avoid foods high in _____.

6. Fluoxetine, one of the first SSRIs approved for use in depression, is also approved for use in women with _____.

7. _____, used as an antidepressant, is also used to aid in smoking cessation.

8. Some of the drawbacks of tricyclic antidepressant therapy are the many _____ effects associated with the drugs, including dry mouth, urinary retention, and constipation.

CHAPTER 22

Psychotherapeutic Agents

■ Matching

Match the following words with the appropriate definition.

1. _____ schizophrenia
2. _____ narcolepsy
3. _____ attention-deficit disorder
4. _____ neuroleptic
5. _____ major tranquilizer
6. _____ mania
7. _____ antipsychotic

A. A state of hyperexcitability

B. Behavioral syndrome characterized by an inability to concentrate

C. A mental disorder characterized by daytime sleepiness and sudden periods of loss of wakefulness

D. Name once used to describe antipsychotic drugs

E. A drug used to treat a disorder of the thought processes; a dopamine receptor blocker

F. A psychotic disorder characterized by delusions, hallucinations, and thought and speech disturbances

G. Antipsychotic drug, so named because of the numerous neurologic adverse effects caused by these drugs

■ Patient Teaching Checklist

Mr. Brown is a landscaper who is busy in the spring and summer. He has been treated for manifestations of a psychotic disorder but has had drug sensitivity reactions to most of the drugs he has tried. The psychiatrist has ordered chlorpromazine, 10 mg orally (PO) every 6 hours (q6h) to try to control his behavior. Mr. Brown is referred to the nurse for drug teaching. Using the patient teaching checklist as a template, prepare a written drug card for Mr. Brown.

■ Web Exercise

Your patient has been diagnosed with seasonal affective disorder (SAD). She does not want to take any medication, although her signs and symptoms are nearly incapacitating. Help your patient investigate alternative treatment plans for SAD. Go to http://www.mhsource.com.

■ Word Scramble

Unscramble the following letters to form the names of some commonly used antipsychotic agents.

1. doennilmo _____

2. zipodime _____

3. sziidpornae _____

4. ttiinhheexo _____

5. presiirodne _____

6. dmaezsionrie _____

7. paxoilen _____

8. oildoperah _____

9. promflutizrien _____

10. noclepazi _____

CHAPTER 23

Antiepileptic Agents

■ Fill in the Blanks

1. _____, the most prevalent of the neurologic disorders, is a collection of different syndromes, all characterized by a sudden discharge of excessive electrical energy from nerve cells located within the brain.

2. Sudden discharge of excessive electrical energy in the brain leads to a(n) _____.

3. If motor nerves are stimulated by this sudden discharge of electrical energy, a _____ may occur with tonic–clonic muscle contractions.

4. Epilepsy is managed using a class of drugs called _____.

5. Tonic–clonic seizures, formerly known as _____, involve dramatic tonic–clonic muscle contractions, loss of consciousness, and a recovery period that is characterized by confusion and exhaustion.

6. A petit mal seizure, now called a(n) _____, involves abrupt, brief (3–5 seconds) periods of loss of consciousness.

7. Seizures that involve short, sporadic periods of muscle contractions that last for several minutes are called _____.

8. Seizures that are related to very high fevers and usually involve convulsions are called _____.

9. The most dangerous of seizure conditions is a state in which seizures rapidly recur again and again, which is referred to as _____.

10. Partial or _____ seizures involve one area of the brain and do not spread throughout the entire brain.

■ Nursing Care Guide

Meghan Smith, a college student, is found beside her car having a tonic–clonic seizure. Safety precautions were taken to avoid injury, and Meghan was transported to the infirmary for evaluation. She has no history of seizure disorders and denies drug or alcohol use. Her parents are called and informed about what happened, and the attending physician starts her on phenytoin (Dilantin) as a precautionary measure until further tests can be done. Meghan's parents have her transported to a hospital near their home. Prepare a nursing care plan to be transported with Meghan. Because she is a healthy young adult with no other known problems, the care plan will reflect drug therapy.

■ Crossword Puzzle

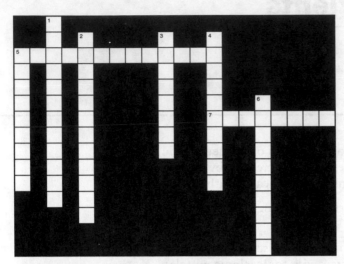

ACROSS

5 Sedative/hypnotic used to treat many forms of seizures

7 Drug of choice for petit mal seizures

DOWN

1 Saved for use in the treatment of petit mal seizures in patients refractory to other agents

2 Used to prevent seizures following neurosurgery

3 Also used to relieve tension and muscle spasm

4 Used to treat petit mal seizures, myoclonic seizures

5 Dilantin

6 Used as an adjunct in treating petit mal seizures

■ Word Search

Circle the following words related to antiepileptic therapy hidden in the following grid. The words may appear diagonally, vertically, or horizontally.

acetazolamide
antiepileptic
carbamazepine
clonazepam
convulsion
diazepam
epilepsy
ethosuximide
ethotoin
felbamate
gabapentin
grand mal
methsuximide
phensuximide
phenytoin
seizure
succinimides
tiagabine
valproic acid
zonisamide

```
D E G I K L O Q S U W E R Y B E S T F R I E N I
A T R S G R A N D M A L E R S H E W W A S M Y V
N E O L O R U V W O E B M E M E R O L U O C I O
I A N T I E P I L E C T I C L O N A Z E P A M M
G O I N E S L E R O E N H I N T A T U O S T H A
I N N H O D I A Z E P A M S T E L L A R L I G C
N O G V N Z I D E D S E I Z U R E S E A G N Z Y
O S U A I X O M R L L S A R E X W D O L F E O E
T U N L M W E P I L E P S Y E T I I R O V N N M
H C I P H E N S U X I M I D E M A M F S Y I I H
S C O R I V I O V L U E T S A W E E I T V B S F
A I T O D E L L I W S S A L W T E L O D I A A Y
D N O I S L U V N O C C O C I N O T Y S E G M P
W I H C O N V U L S I Z O H N E P I L E P A I M
I M T A E P D N A T A L A S T U X E D I B I D J
N I E C P P E R T T A R R A F E L B A M A T E O
O D A I L A P H E N Y T O I N P S Y N A P S O R
L E S D A W D C A R B A M A Z E P I N E O R M A
C S A U L G A B A P E N T I N E O T R O C K I N
H X O T I W O G O T H G I T N I N A M R E P V S
```

CHAPTER 24

Antiparkinsonism Agents

■ Fill in the Blanks

Label the following diagram, indicating the interrelationship of neurons that leads to Parkinson's disease.

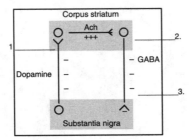

■ Word Scramble

Unscramble the following letters to form the names of commonly used antiparkinsonism drugs.

1. poolaved _____

2. yopclicdinre _____

3. gloierped _____

4. pedrinibe _____

5. tanmadaeni _____

6. poorinirel _____

7. zoptrebnine _____

8. inetripcoromb _____

■ Web Exercise

M. J. was diagnosed with Parkinson's disease at the age of 42, when tremors began to interfere with his job as a watch repairman. He was well controlled on carbidopa–levodopa (Sinemet) for 7 years, but now the disease is progressing rapidly. You are trying to work with the family to prepare them for what is to come and to help them to make the most of M. J.'s abilities while they struggle with his prognosis. Go to http://www.ninds.nih.gov and find information that will be helpful for this family.

■ Multiple Choice

Select the best answer to the following.

1. Parkinson's disease is characterized by:
   a. increased salivation.
   b. a lack of coordination.
   c. loss of memory.
   d. a history of head injury.

2. Although the actual cause is not known, it is known that people with Parkinson's disease lose:
   a. acetylcholine-producing cells in the corpus striatum.
   b. GABA-producing cells in the basal ganglia.
   c. acetylcholine-producing cells in the basal ganglia.
   d. dopamine-producing cells in the substantia nigra.

3. Patients with Parkinson's disease need to know that:
   a. the disease is easily cured.
   b. the disease can often be cured surgically.
   c. the disease is progressive and debilitating.
   d. a combination of various drugs can prevent the progress of the disease.

4. Drug therapy in Parkinson's disease is aimed at:
   a. increasing dopamine levels and blocking acetylcholine effects.
   b. increasing acetylcholine effects and blocking γ-aminobutyric acid (GABA) receptors.
   c. increasing GABA effects and blocking dopamine.
   d. increasing dopamine levels and increasing acetylcholine effects.

5. Patients receiving anticholinergic drugs to treat Parkinson's disease must be monitored for:
   a. decreased heart rate and increased blood pressure.
   b. diarrhea and fluid imbalance.
   c. dry mouth and urinary retention.
   d. increased sweating and flushing.

6. To prevent adverse effects, levodopa is given in combination with:
   a. atropine.
   b. carbidopa.
   c. vitamin B_6.
   d. phenothiazines.

7. Pergolide and ropinirole act to:
   a. increase the levels of dopamine at the receptor site.
   b. stimulate the release of more dopamine from the nerve endings.
   c. block the reuptake of dopamine at the nerve ending.
   d. directly stimulate the dopamine receptors.

8. There is a serious risk of hypertensive crisis if dopaminergic drugs are taken with:

    a. monoamine oxidase (MAO) inhibitors.

    b. tricyclic antidepressants.

    c. anticholinergic drugs.

    d. antihistamines.

CHAPTER 25

Muscle Relaxants

■ Matching

Match the following words with the appropriate definitions.

1. _____ spasticity
2. _____ hypertonia
3. _____ hypotonia
4. _____ basal ganglia
5. _____ intraneurons
6. _____ pyramidal tract
7. _____ extrapyramidal tract
8. _____ cerebellum

A. Neurons that communicate between other neurons
B. Fibers within the central nervous system (CNS) that control precise, intentional movement
C. Sustained contractions of muscles
D. Lower portion of the brain associated with coordination of muscle movements and voluntary muscle movement
E. State of excessive muscle response and activity
F. Lower area of the brain associated with coordination of unconscious muscle movements
G. Cells that coordinate unconsciously controlled muscle activity
H. State of limited or absent muscle response and activity

■ Fill in the Blanks

Label the parts of the nerve and muscle reflex.

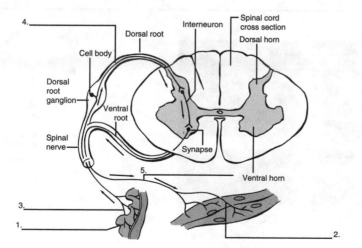

■ True or False

Indicate whether the following statements are true (T) or false (F).

_____ 1. The nerves that affect movement, position, and posture are the spinal sensory neurons.

_____ 2. The basal ganglia and the cerebellum modulate spinal motor nerve activity and help coordinate activity between various muscle groups.

_____ 3. Fibers that control precise, intentional movement make up the extrapyramidal tract.

_____ 4. The pyramidal tract modulates or coordinates unconsciously controlled muscle activity and allows the body to make automatic adjustments in posture, position, and balance.

_____ 5. Muscle spasticity is the result of damage to neurons within the CNS rather than injury to peripheral structures.

_____ 6. Excessive stimulation of muscles is referred to as hypotonia.

_____ 7. Centrally acting skeletal muscle relaxants work in the CNS to interfere with the reflexes that are causing the muscle spasm.

_____ 8. Dantrolene acts within skeletal muscle fibers, interfering with the release of potassium from the muscle tubules, to prevent the fibers from contracting.

_____ 9. The primary indication for the use of centrally acting skeletal muscle agents is the relief of discomfort associated with acute, painful musculoskeletal conditions.

_____ 10. Centrally acting muscle relaxants should be used as an adjunct to rest, physical therapy, and other measures.

■ Crossword Puzzle

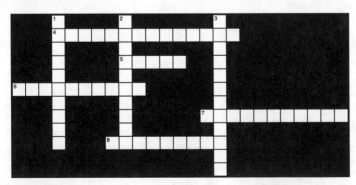

ACROSS

2 Coordinates unconsciously controlled muscle activity

5 Relaxation and contraction of a muscle group

6 State of excessive muscle response and activity

7 Nerve cell that communicates with other nerves

8 Fibers that control precise, intentional movement

DOWN

1 Large lower area of the brain

2 Sustained muscle contraction

3 Lower area of the brain associated with coordination

CHAPTER 26

Narcotics and Antimigraine Agents

■ Word Search

Circle the names of the following frequently used narcotics hidden in the following grid. Words may appear horizontally, vertically, or diagonally.

alfentanil
codeine
fentanyl
hydrocodone
hydromorphone
levorphanol
meperidine
methadone
morphine
oxycodone
oxymorphone
propoxyphene
sufentanil

A	S	T	E	O	X	Y	M	O	R	P	H	O	N	E	P	R	O
E	N	I	D	I	R	E	P	E	M	H	E	N	O	N	R	T	L
E	E	O	E	L	N	P	E	M	E	L	N	O	R	O	O	O	L
N	A	N	P	I	O	S	N	N	H	I	Y	M	S	D	P	L	I
O	D	S	E	O	P	H	E	N	T	I	O	N	G	A	O	X	N
D	I	D	O	P	J	H	N	I	H	O	T	R	A	H	X	I	A
O	O	R	A	H	I	L	O	T	A	N	R	I	M	T	Y	L	T
C	N	E	M	O	X	Y	C	O	D	O	N	E	S	E	P	O	N
O	X	Y	M	O	P	H	N	I	O	R	I	N	S	M	H	E	E
R	Y	N	M	O	R	P	H	I	N	E	C	O	Q	A	E	L	F
D	O	R	U	L	I	P	Y	S	U	F	E	N	T	A	N	I	L
Y	L	E	V	O	R	P	H	A	N	O	L	C	H	L	E	M	A
H	Y	D	R	O	M	O	R	P	H	O	N	E	I	O	N	R	I
D	E	P	R	U	N	L	Y	N	A	T	N	X	E	T	Y	S	T

■ Matching

Match the generic name of these commonly used narcotic agonists with the associated brand name.

1. _____ fentanyl
2. _____ hydrocodone
3. _____ hydromorphone
4. _____ levomethadyl
5. _____ levorphanol
6. _____ meperidine
7. _____ methadone
8. _____ morphine
9. _____ oxycodone
10. _____ propoxyphene

A. *Darvon*
B. *Dolophine*
C. *Demerol*
D. *Dilaudid*
E. *OxyContin*
F. *Hycodan*
G. *Duragesic*
H. *ORLAAM*
I. *Roxanol*
J. *Levo-Dromoran*

■ Multiple Choice

Select the best answer to the following.

1. The term *migraine headache* is used to describe several different types of syndromes, all of which include:
   a. severe, throbbing headaches on one side of the head.
   b. blinding headaches in the frontal lobe.
   c. loss of consciousness.
   d. the presence of an anticipatory aura.

2. Cluster headaches:
   a. are frequently occurring migraine headaches.
   b. start during sleep and involve sharp, steady eye pain lasting for 15 to 90 minutes with sweating, flushing, tearing, and nasal congestion.
   c. occur in conjunction with airborne allergies.
   d. are tension headaches.

3. Tension headaches:
   a. are migraine headaches.
   b. usually occur during stress and feel like a dull band around the entire head.
   c. last for up to 2 hours.
   d. are cluster headaches.

4. Ergot derivatives are used to treat migraines because they:
   a. are not associated with any adverse effects.
   b. are inexpensive because they come from molds.
   c. cause constriction of cranial blood vessels, decreasing the pulsation of cranial arteries and decreasing the hyperperfusion of the basilar artery vascular bed.
   d. are slow acting and have prolonged effects.

5. The triptans are a group of drugs that:
   a. bind to selective serotonin receptor sites to cause vasoconstriction of cranial vessels, relieving the signs and symptoms of migraine headache.
   b. must be delivered by injection.
   c. have many more adverse effects than the ergot derivatives.
   d. can be safely used in the elderly and patients with known vascular disease.

■ Definitions

Define the following terms.

1. A fibers _____

   _____

2. A-delta and C fibers _____

   _____

3. gate-control theory _____

_____

4. migraine headache _____

_____

5. narcotics _____

_____

6. narcotic agonists _____

_____

7. narcotic agonists–antagonists _____

_____

8. narcotic antagonists _____

_____

9. opioid receptors _____

_____

10. triptan _____

_____

CHAPTER 27

General and Local Anesthetic Agents

■ Fill in the Blanks

Describe what occurs at each of the four stages of anesthesia.

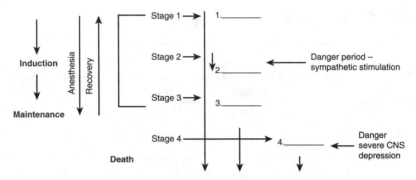

■ Nursing Care Guide

Lorne Perkins, a 26-year-old football player, is admitted to your short-term surgery unit for repair of an inguinal hernia. He has elected to have a spinal anesthetic for the surgery. Prepare a nursing care guide that will follow him to the recovery area after surgery.

■ Fill in the Blanks

1. General anesthetics are drugs used to produce _____, _____, _____, and _____ and to block muscle reflexes that could interfere with a surgical procedure or put the patient at risk for harm.

2. Anesthesia proceeds through predictable stages from _____ to total central nervous system (CNS) depression and _____.

3. _____ is the time from the beginning of anesthesia administration until the patient reaches surgical anesthesia.

4. _____ involves giving a variety of drugs, including anticholinergics, rapid intravenous (IV) anesthetics, inhaled anesthetics, neuromuscular junction (NMJ) blockers, and narcotics.

5. Local anesthetics block the _____, preventing the transmission of pain sensations and motor stimuli.

6. The use of general anesthetics involves a widespread _____ that could be harmful, especially in patients with underlying CNS, cardiovascular (CV), or respiratory diseases.

7. Patients receiving general anesthetics should be monitored for any adverse effects, offered reassurance, and provided with safety precautions until the recovery of _____, _____, and _____.

8. The adverse effects of local anesthetics may be related to their local blocking of sensation; such effects may include _____, _____, and _____.

■ Word Search

Circle the following anesthesia-related words hidden in the following grid. Words may appear diagonally, vertically, or horizontally.

amnesia
analgesia
balanced
benzocaine
butamben
enflurane
etidocaine
gases
general
halothane
induction
isoflurane
ketamine
local
mepivacaine
midazolam
procaine
propofol
unconsciousness
volatile

C	I	D	E	R	O	C	H	A	D	O	N	A	Y	M	O	R	A	I	N
E	C	A	M	I	D	A	Z	O	L	A	M	F	T	A	F	A	S	L	E
B	B	A	E	I	L	S	E	Y	I	S	O	F	L	U	R	A	N	E	P
H	E	C	P	P	R	E	E	M	L	A	R	E	N	E	G	S	L	E	A
U	N	C	I	R	K	S	J	O	H	N	A	S	O	N	S	D	A	T	N
R	Z	E	V	O	L	A	T	I	L	E	B	M	M	E	A	Y	E	I	L
M	O	E	A	P	O	G	R	R	N	I	S	O	N	N	D	A	R	D	T
I	C	N	C	O	R	R	O	M	R	D	E	S	D	E	A	V	B	O	H
S	A	A	A	F	O	N	C	U	L	D	U	D	L	E	S	S	A	C	P
S	I	H	I	O	I	R	R	O	M	O	E	C	I	K	N	I	L	A	V
O	N	T	N	L	A	N	P	E	I	P	C	P	T	E	R	G	A	I	E
O	E	O	E	R	A	I	D	C	E	C	G	A	O	I	Z	T	N	N	R
L	M	L	Z	O	G	C	S	H	O	P	S	B	L	U	O	S	C	E	T
R	E	A	I	S	S	N	A	E	L	P	R	O	C	A	I	N	E	R	E
I	N	H	T	I	O	N	L	A	G	D	Y	T	R	A	M	P	D	A	S
S	O	P	M	C	I	S	E	N	F	L	U	R	A	N	E	M	E	A	T
G	T	R	N	I	L	N	X	K	E	T	A	M	I	N	E	A	N	D	E
I	B	U	O	L	B	U	T	A	M	B	E	N	I	T	U	A	T	E	V
P	E	U	S	E	V	O	S	A	N	S	H	J	A	E	L	J	H	J	E
Y	L	L	T	N	W	P	E	O	N	O	B	O	R	F	M	I	O	R	R

CHAPTER 28

Neuromuscular Junction Blocking Agents

■ Fill in the Blanks

Indicate the actions and functions of the neuromuscular junction (NMJ) and the sliding filament theory of muscle contraction.

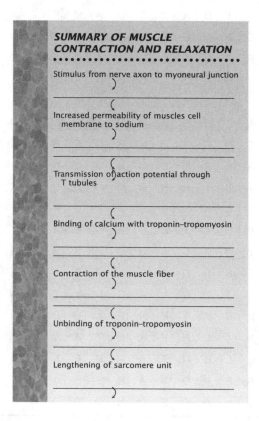

SUMMARY OF MUSCLE CONTRACTION AND RELAXATION

Stimulus from nerve axon to myoneural junction

_____

Increased permeability of muscles cell membrane to sodium

_____

Transmission of action potential through T tubules

_____

Binding of calcium with troponin–tropomyosin

_____

Contraction of the muscle fiber

_____

Unbinding of troponin–tropomyosin

_____

Lengthening of sarcomere unit

_____

■ Crossword Puzzle

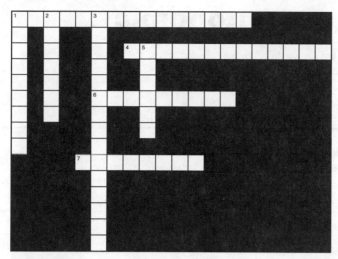

ACROSS

1 Depolarizing neuromuscular junction blocker
4 Neurotransmitter at the neuromuscular junction
6 Loss of muscle function
7 Prevents the formation of actinomyosin bridges

3 Preventing, not causing, cell depolarization
5 Poison used on the tips of arrows and spears

DOWN

1 Functional unit of a muscle
2 Ion needed for muscle contraction

■ Matching

Match the NMJ blocker with the appropriate brand name.

1. _____ atracurium
2. _____ cisatracurium
3. _____ doxacurium
4. _____ mivacurium
5. _____ pancuronium
6. _____ pipecuronium
7. _____ rocuronium
8. _____ vecuronium

A. *Arduan*
B. *Tracrium*
C. *Norcuron*
D. *Nuromax*
E. *Nimbex*
F. *Mivacron*
G. *Zemuron*
H. *Pavulon*

CHAPTER 29

Introduction to the Autonomic Nervous System

■ Fill in the Blanks

Fill in the following table describing the characteristics of the sympathetic and parasympathetic branches of the autonomic nervous system

COMPARISON OF THE SYMPATHETIC AND PARASYMPATHETIC NERVOUS SYSTEMS

Characteristic	Sympathetic	Parasympathetic
CNS nerve origin		
Preganglionic neuron		
Preganglionic neurotransmitter		
Ganglia location		
Postganglionic neuron		
Postganglionic neurotransmitter		
Neurotransmitter terminator		
General response		

■ Matching

Match the following words with the appropriate definition.

1. _____ autonomic nervous system
2. _____ sympathetic nervous system
3. _____ parasympathetic nervous system
4. _____ ganglia
5. _____ adrenergic receptors
6. _____ cholinergic receptors
7. _____ β-receptors
8. _____ α-receptors
9. _____ muscarinic receptors
10. _____ nicotinic receptors
11. _____ acetylcholinesterase
12. _____ monoamine oxidase (MAO)

A. Adrenergic receptors that are found in smooth muscles
B. Closely packed group of nerve cell bodies
C. "Fight-or-flight" response mediator
D. Enzyme that breaks down norepinephrine
E. Cholinergic receptors that also respond to stimulation by nicotine
F. "Rest-and-digest" response mediator
G. Receptor sites on effectors that respond to acetylcholine
H. Adrenergic receptors found in the heart, lungs, and vascular smooth muscle
I. Receptor sites on effectors that respond to norepinephrine
J. Cholinergic receptors that also respond to stimulation by muscarine

K. Portion of the central and peripheral nervous systems that, with the endocrine system, functions to maintain internal homeostasis

L. Enzyme that deactivates acetylcholine released from the nerve axon

■ Fill in the Blanks

Fill in the following chart, which shows the effects of the sympathetic and parasympathetic systems on the body's organ system. Insert the specific sympathetic receptor type in column 3 as appropriate.

EFFECTS OF AUTONOMIC STIMULATION

Effector Site	Sympathetic Reaction	Receptor	Parasympathetic Reaction
Heart			
Blood vessels			
Skin, mucous membranes			
Skeletal muscle			
Bronchial muscle			
GI System			
Muscle motility and tone			
Sphincters			
Secretions			
Salivary glands			
Gallbladder			
Liver			
Urinary bladder			
Detrusor muscle			
Trigone muscle and sphincter			
Eye structures			
Iris radial muscle			
Iris sphincter muscle			
Ciliary muscle			
Lacrimal glands			
Skin structures			
Sweat glands			
Piloerector muscles			
Sex organs			
Male			
Female			

■ Word Search

Circle the following words related to the autonomic nervous system hidden in the following grid. Words may appear diagonally, vertically, or horizontally.

acetylcholine
acetylcholinesterase
adrenergic
alpha receptor
autonomic
beta receptor
bronchodilation
cholinergic
fight
flight
ganglia
monoamine oxidase
muscarinic
nicotinic
norepinephrine
parasympathetic
piloerection
sympathetic

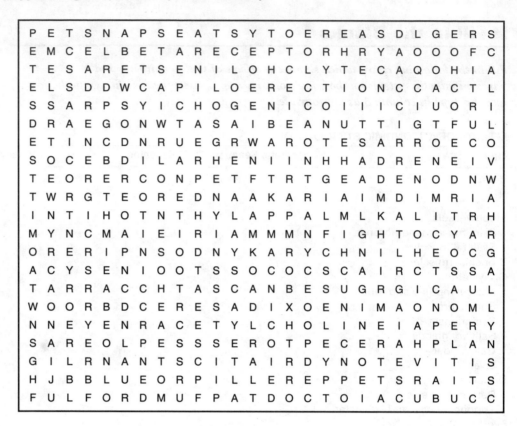

```
P E T S N A P S E A T S Y T O E R E A S D L G E R S
E M C E L B E T A R E C E P T O R H R Y A O O O F C
T E S A R E T S E N I L O H C L Y T E C A Q O H I A
E L S D D W C A P I L O E R E C T I O N C C A C T L
S S A R P S Y I C H O G E N I C O I I I C I U O R I
D R A E G O N W T A S A I B E A N U T T I G T F U L
E T I N C D N R U E G R W A R O T E S A R R O E C O
S O C E B D I L A R H E N I I N H H A D R E N E I V
T E O R E R C O N P E T F T R T G E A D E N O D N W
T W R G T E O R E D N A A K A R I A I M D I M R I A
I N T I H O T N T H Y L A P P A L M L K A L I T R H
M Y N C M A I E I R I A M M M N F I G H T O C Y A R
O R E R I P N S O D N Y K A R Y C H N I L H E O C G
A C Y S E N I O O T S S O C O C S C A I R C T S S A
T A R R A C C H T A S C A N B E S U G R G I C A U L
W O O R B D C E R E S A D I X O E N I M A O N O M L
N N E Y E N R A C E T Y L C H O L I N E I A P E R Y
S A R E O L P E S S S E R O T P E C E R A H P L A N
G I L R N A N T S C I T A I R D Y N O T E V I T I S
H J B B L U E O R P I L L E R E P P E T S R A I T S
F U L F O R D M U F P A T D O C T O I A C U B U C C
```

CHAPTER 30

Adrenergic Agents

■ Multiple Choice

Select the best answer to the following.

1. Adrenergic agonists are:
   a. drugs used to stimulate the cholinergic receptors within the sympathetic nervous system (SNS).
   b. also called sympathomimetic drugs.
   c. drugs used to block the effects of the SNS.
   d. used to treat hypertension.

2. α- and β-adrenergic agonists:
   a. stimulate all of the adrenergic receptors in the SNS.
   b. are used to prevent a fight-or-flight response.
   c. are most useful in treating hypertension.
   d. are associated with few adverse effects.

3. Clonidine:
   a. is a β-specific adrenergic agonist.
   b. is used to treat shock.
   c. stimulates α_2-receptors and blocks norepinephrine release from nerve axons.
   d. may be useful in treating asthma.

4. β_2-specific adrenergic agonists are:
   a. used to manage and treat asthma, bronchospasm, and other obstructive pulmonary diseases.
   b. used to stimulate bronchoconstriction.
   c. not associated with any cardiovascular effects.
   d. useful for stimulating labor.

5. Isoproterenol, a β-agonist:
   a. is used to treat hypertension.
   b. can be used to treat arrhythmias and also to treat bronchospasm and asthma.
   c. can only be given parenterally.
   d. blocks the effects of the SNS on the heart.

6. Ephedrine is a rather toxic adrenergic agonist, which is now primarily used:
   a. for shock.
   b. as a nasal decongestant.
   c. to slow rapid heart rates.
   d. to stimulate the heart during cardiac arrest.

7. The use of adrenergic agonists is contraindicated with:
   a. glaucoma.
   b. respiratory distress.
   c. pheochromocytoma.
   d. hypotension.

8. The sympathomimetic drug that would be the drug of choice for treating shock and hypotension is:
   a. ephedrine.
   b. norepinephrine.
   c. metaraminol.
   d. dopamine.

9. The β-agonist that is used to manage preterm labor is:
   a. epinephrine.
   b. ritodrine.
   c. ephedrine.
   d. isoproterenol.

10. β-agonists that are specifically used to treat bronchospasm and asthma do not include:
    a. salmeterol.
    b. isoproterenol.
    c. albuterol.
    d. bitolterol.

■ Word Scramble

Unscramble the following letters to form the names of frequently used adrenergic agonists.

1. redhepnie _____
2. indocline _____
3. modanpie _____
4. torridine _____
5. aboutdimen _____
6. repronininehep _____
7. ratammnolie _____
8. yepphhnneeirl _____
9. nineppehire _____
10. pontlioreesor _____

■ Fill in the Blanks

Insert the α-adrenergic drugs discussed in this chapter at their appropriate sites of action.

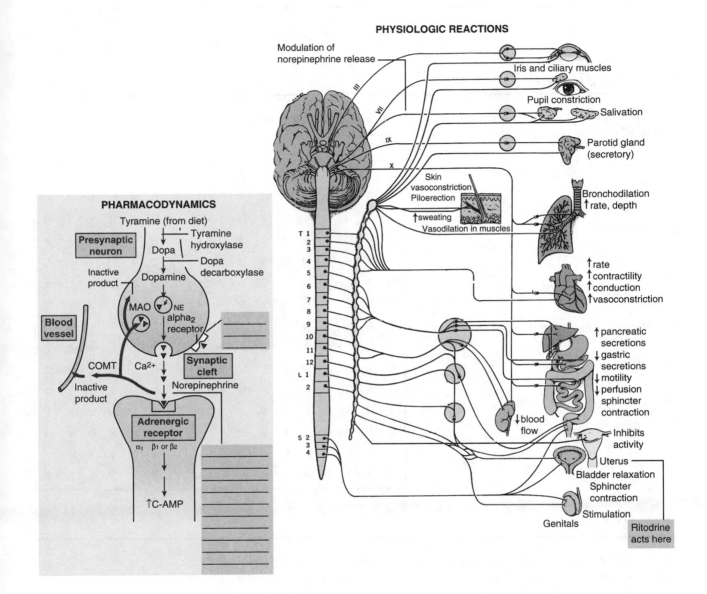

PHYSIOLOGIC REACTIONS

CHAPTER 31

Adrenergic Blocking Agents

■ Word Search

Circle the following names of adrenergic blocking agents hidden in the following grid. Words may appear diagonally, vertically, or horizontally.

atenolol
bisoprolol
carteolol
esmolol
guanadrel
labetalol
metoprolol
nadolol
phenoxybenzamine
pindolol
prazosin
sotalol
terazosin
timolol

```
L K U I N O Z A S O N A C E T A C
I O B M O R T X I T E C A M H A D
B I B P I N D O L O L H R E E T H
L P M E N I O Z I L L E T S O E P
C P H E N O X Y B E N Z A M I N E
H X Y S A Z O S I N I O S O L O X
O X Y P R A Z O S I N N H L Y L G
Z A S I N O O X C A R T E O L O L
T E R A Z O S I N M L Y L L I L Z
M I R R O B I S O P R O L O L I E
O S G U A N A D R E L L L Y X Z B
T H H R A S N I N A D O L O L A F
H I R O L A B E T A L O L X M Y W
O M E T O P R O L O L K L Y S I O
P P T O P H S L L M Y Y O Z A S T
```

■ Web Exercise

Your patient has been diagnosed with essential hypertension. Because his father died at a young age from a heart attack, he is concerned about his risk of developing heart disease and asks you for more information. Go to the Internet and develop a teaching packet to address his concerns.

■ True or False

Indicate whether the following statements are true (T) or false (F).

_____ 1. Adrenergic blocking agents are also called sympathomimetic drugs.

_____ 2. Drugs that block all adrenergic receptors are primarily used to treat cardiac-related conditions.

_____ 3. Adrenergic blocking agents competitively block the effects of norepinephrine at both α- and β-receptors throughout the sympathetic nervous system (SNS), causing the signs and symptoms associated with a sympathetic stress reaction.

_____ 4. The adverse effects associated with adrenergic blocking agents of cardiac arrhythmias, hypotension, congestive heart failure, pulmonary edema, cerebral vascular accident, or stroke are related to the lack of stimulatory effects and loss of vascular tone in the cardiovascular system.

_____ 5. The therapeutic effects of the α_1-selective adrenergic blocking agents come from their ability to block the postsynaptic α_1-receptor sites. This causes a decrease in vascular tone and vasodilation, which leads to a fall in blood pressure.

_____ 6. The β-adrenergic blocking agents are used to treat asthma and obstructive pulmonary diseases.

_____ 7. Propranolol is a widely prescribed drug that has been used to treat migraine headaches and stage fright (situational anxiety).

_____ 8. β-adrenergic blocking agents should not be stopped abruptly after chronic therapy but should be tapered gradually over 2 weeks.

■ Matching

Match each of the following adrenergic blockers with the commonly used brand name associated with it.

1. _____ metoprolol
2. _____ esmolol
3. _____ atenolol
4. _____ carvedilol
5. _____ bisoprolol
6. _____ acebutolol
7. _____ timolol
8. _____ propranolol
9. _____ doxazosin
10. _____ nadolol
11. _____ prazosin
12. _____ sotalol

A. *Cardura*
B. *Blocadren*
C. *Betapace*
D. *Lopressor*
E. *Coreg*
F. *Minipress*
G. *Inderal*
H. *Sectral*
I. *Brevibloc*
J. *Zebeta*
K. *Tenormin*
L. *Corgard*

CHAPTER 32

Cholinergic Agents

■ Fill in the Blanks

Fill in the pertinent information regarding the cholinergic receptor site and indicate where direct acting and indirect acting cholinergic agonists work.

PHYSIOLOGIC RESPONSES TO CHOLINERGIC DRUGS

ACh receptors in cortex aid memory learning

Constrictor

Dilator

Ciliary ganglion — Lens accommodation

Sphenopalatine ganglion — Pupil constriction

Submandibular ganglion — ↑ lacrimal secretions

Otic ganglion — ↑ salivation

Parotid gland (secretory)

Sweating — Motor

↓ synaptate effect
↑ secretions

Inhibitory — ↓ rate ↓ contractility ↓ conduction

Celiac ganglion

↑ secretions
↑ motility
↓ sphincter constriction

Muscle contraction
Sphincter relaxation

Uterus

Pelvic nerve

Inhibitory
Motor

Motor

Vasodilation

Genitals

PHARMACODYNAMICS OF CHOLINERGIC DRUGS

Resection of cholinergic nerve terminal

Nerve terminal

Acetyl CoA
+
Choline (from diet) — Enzyme
ACh

Blood vessel

Choline
+
Acetic acid

Ca2+
ACh — Acetycholinesterase

Muscarinic or nicotinic cholinergic receptor

Neuron or effector cell

Neuromuscular junction; causes muscle contraction

■ Crossword Puzzle

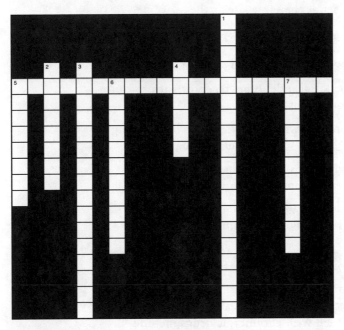

ACROSS

5 Enzyme responsible for the break down of acetylcholine

DOWN

1 Mimicking the effects of the parasympathetic nervous system

2 Irreversible acetylcholinesterase inhibitor used in warfare

3 Autoimmune disorder characterized by destruction of receptor sites

4 Constriction of the pupils

5 Drugs that increase effects or activity

6 Responding to acetylcholine

7 Degenerative disease of the cortex with loss of acetylcholine-producing cells

■ Matching

Match the drug with its usual indication. (Some drugs may have more than one indication.)

1. _____ pilocarpine

2. _____ tacrine

3. _____ neostigmine

4. _____ ambenonium

5. _____ pyridostigmine

6. _____ edrophonium

7. _____ rivastigmine

8. _____ donepezil

A. Diagnosis of myasthenia gravis

B. Treatment of myasthenia gravis

C. Antidote for neuromuscular junction (NMJ) blockers

D. Glaucoma, miosis

E. Alzheimer's disease

■ Fill in the Blanks

1. Cholinergic drugs are chemicals that act at the same site as the neurotransmitter _____.

2. Cholinergic drugs are often also called _____ drugs because their action mimics the action of the parasympathetic nervous system.

3. _____ cholinergic drugs act at acetylcholine receptor sites to cause the same reaction as acetylcholine would cause.

4. Cholinergic agents that prevent the breakdown of acetylcholine by blocking acetylcholinesterase are called _____ cholinergic drugs.

5. _____ is a progressive neurological condition that is marked by loss of the acetylcholine-producing neurons in the cerebral cortex.

6. _____ _____ is a chronic muscular disease that is caused by a defect in neuromuscular transmission; cholinergic drugs help patients with this disease.

7. Common adverse effects in the gastrointestinal (GI) tract seen with cholinergic drugs include _____, _____, _____, and _____.

8. Cardiovascular effects that are often seen with cholinergic drugs include _____, _____, and _____.

CHAPTER 33

Anticholinergic Agents

■ Fill in the Blanks

Fill in the following table with the effects of anticholinergic agents.

Physiological Effect	Therapeutic Use
Gastrointestinal (GI) tract	
Smooth muscle	
Secretory glands	
Urinary tract	
Biliary tract	
Bronchial muscle	
Cardiovascular system	
Ocular effects	
Secretions	
Central nervous system (CNS)	

■ Patient Teaching Checklist

E. S. is a 60-year-old bread deliveryman with mild prostatic hypertrophy. He is seen in the clinic for recurring bouts of irritable bowel syndrome, which make his job difficult. He is to be started on dicyclomine and will need teaching information. Prepare a drug teaching card for E. S. to take with him when he leaves the clinic.

■ Fill in the Blanks

1. Anticholinergic drugs block the effects of _____ at cholinergic receptor sites.

2. Anticholinergic drugs are also called _____ drugs because they block the effects of the parasympathetic nervous system.

3. Blocking the parasympathetic system causes the following effects: _____ in heart rate, _____ in GI activity and in urinary bladder tone and function, pupil dilation, and cycloplegia.

4. These drugs also block cholinergic receptors in the CNS and those sympathetic postganglionic cholinergic receptors, including those that cause _____.

5. _____ is the prevention of accommodation of the lens for near vision.

6. Relaxation of the pupil of the eye is called a(n) _____ effect.

7. _____ is the most commonly used anticholinergic drug.

8. Patients receiving anticholinergic drugs must be monitored for problems related to eating because of the adverse effects of _____ and _____ .

■ Crossword Puzzle

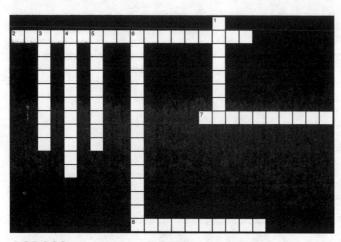

ACROSS

2 Blocking the effects of the parasympathetic nervous system

7 Anticholinergic drug used to dilate pupils during certain fashion stages

8 Inability of the lens of the eye to accommodate for near vision

DOWN

1 Drug frequently used as an anticholinergic drug

3 Holding, urinary retention occurs with the use of these drugs

4 Anticholinergic very effective in treating motion sickness

5 Pupil dilation

6 Drug that opposes the effects of acetylcholine

CHAPTER 34

Introduction to the Endocrine System

■ Fill in the Blanks

Fill in the names of the endocrine glands and their hormones in the following diagram of the traditional endocrine system.

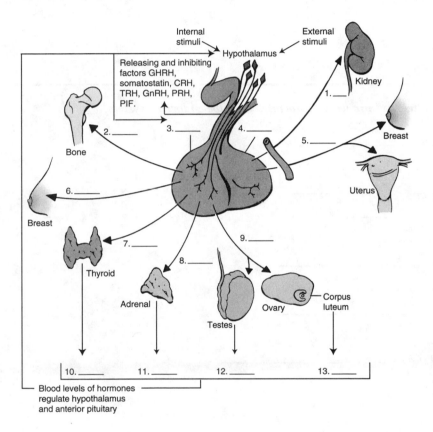

■ Listing

List the five characteristics of a hormone. All hormones:

1. _____

2. _____

3. _____

4. _____

5. _____

■ Matching

Match the anterior pituitary hormone with the endocrine response it elicits.

1. _____ adrenocorticotropic hormone (ACTH)
2. _____ growth hormone (GH)
3. _____ prolactin (PRL)
4. _____ thyroid-stimulating hormone (TSH)
5. _____ follicle-stimulating hormone (FSH)
6. _____ luteinizing hormone (LH)
7. _____ melanocyte-stimulating hormone (MSH)
8. _____ lipoproteins

A. Production of thyroid hormone
B. Stimulation of fat mobilization
C. Stimulation of ovulation
D. Release of cortisol, aldosterone
E. Nerve growth and development
F. Milk production in the mammary glands
G. Simulation of follicle development in the ovaries
H. Protein catabolism and cell growth

■ Word Scramble

Unscramble the following letters to form words associated with the endocrine system.

1. iittuprya dlang _____
2. nurliad yhhtmr _____
3. sleearngi ctasrof _____
4. nniusil _____
5. asumhatlpoyh _____
6. giveanet beefckad _____
7. smorenoh _____
8. torriesop iittuprya _____
9. canparse _____
10. potyhalamhci -ttipuayr sixa _____

CHAPTER 35

Hypothalamic and Pituitary Agents

■ Matching

Match the hypothalamic releasing or inhibiting factor with the corresponding pituitary hormones that are released or inhibited by their stimulation.

1. _____ growth hormone-releasing hormone (GHRH)
2. _____ thyrotropin-releasing hormone (TRH)
3. _____ gonadotropin-releasing hormone (GnRH)
4. _____ corticotropin-releasing factor (CRF)
5. _____ prolactin-releasing factor (PRF)
6. _____ prolactin-inhibiting factor (PIF)
7. _____ somatostatin

A. Release of adrenocorticotrophic hormone (ACTH)
B. Release of follicle-stimulating hormone (FSH) and luteinizing hormone (LH)
C. Inhibition of growth hormone release
D. Release of prolactin
E. Inhibition of prolactin release
F. Release of growth hormone
G. Release of thyroid-stimulating hormone (TSH)

■ Web Exercise

You have been asked to present an inservice to staff of the pediatric endocrine unit, where you are doing your current rotation, about the use of growth hormone for treatment of Turner's syndrome and small stature. You want to ensure that your information is current because this presentation represents 25% of your grade. Go to the Internet to research current information.

■ Matching

Match the drug with its usual indication.

1. _____ CRF
2. _____ nafarelin
3. _____ cosyntropin
4. _____ somatrem
5. _____ goserelin
6. _____ histrelin
7. _____ leuprolide
8. _____ menotropins

A. Treatment of children with growth failure
B. Treatment of specific cancers, endometriosis
C. Diagnosis of Cushing's disease
D. Treatment of prostatic cancers
E. Treatment of precocious puberty, endometriosis
F. Stimulation of ovulation and spermatogenesis
G. Diagnosis of adrenal failure
H. Treatment of precocious puberty

■ WORD SEARCH

Circle the words related to hypothalamic/pituitary hormones hidden in the following grid. Words may appear diagonally, vertically, or horizontally.

acromegaly
bromocriptine
corticotropin
cosyntropin
diabetes insipidus
dwarfism
gigantism
gonadorelin
goserelin
hypopituitarism
leuprolide
lypressin
menotropins
nafarelin
octreotide
protirelin
somatrem
somatropin
vasopressin

N	S	I	R	S	D	N	H	T	I	O	G	N	R	C	D	N	E	R	A	E	R
O	O	E	E	B	R	O	M	O	C	R	I	P	T	I	N	E	O	L	M	L	I
O	M	D	N	O	O	A	H	T	W	R	M	E	R	T	A	M	O	S	E	S	S
G	E	I	I	T	C	O	S	Y	N	T	R	O	P	I	N	F	I	U	N	E	I
O	N	T	S	A	T	C	P	E	L	M	O	L	S	I	T	R	V	L	O	R	O
T	S	O	S	F	B	I	N	U	S	P	N	A	T	F	A	O	A	T	T	N	N
O	A	E	E	L	H	E	C	I	L	I	L	E	G	T	C	T	S	S	R	I	N
A	E	R	R	E	A	S	T	H	L	F	I	B	I	A	R	O	O	I	O	L	A
E	S	T	P	S	T	N	E	E	O	M	L	U	L	N	O	P	P	N	P	E	S
R	N	C	Y	M	A	A	R	R	S	B	T	L	A	O	M	S	R	I	I	R	O
E	I	O	L	G	I	A	S	I	O	I	L	I	N	N	E	T	E	P	N	I	F
T	L	L	I	Y	F	G	F	T	P	L	N	W	C	E	G	H	S	O	S	T	I
O	E	G	E	A	C	R	A	O	E	E	S	S	I	E	A	E	S	R	N	O	L
N	R	E	N	R	A	N	P	A	V	M	O	T	I	S	L	A	I	T	A	R	E
O	E	N	P	W	O	Y	S	H	M	O	S	I	S	P	Y	M	N	A	I	P	N
D	S	O	D	T	H	Y	T	O	T	R	O	P	I	N	I	P	O	M	L	A	D
S	O	L	I	C	L	E	U	P	R	O	L	I	D	E	R	D	E	O	X	E	N
E	G	O	A	D	L	N	I	L	E	R	O	D	A	N	O	G	U	S	O	I	T
M	T	C	O	R	T	I	C	O	T	R	O	P	I	N	N	B	U	S	T	W	I
I	Y	S	M	N	R	A	I	Y	H	C	C	E	E	H	T	T	U	O	H	I	T

Adrenocortical Agents

■ Word Scramble

Unscramble the following letters to form the names of adrenocortical agents.

1. sonnderpie _____

2. toolninemacir _____

3. sothatobeemen _____

4. coorsdyrthinoe _____

5. soddubenie _____

6. solidefunlie _____

7. sorticone _____

8. mexdateshoen _____

■ Crossword Puzzle

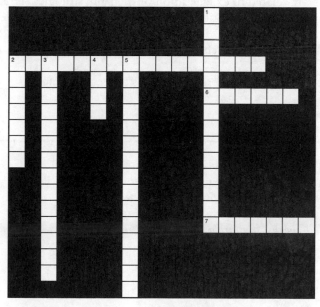

ACROSS

2 Steroid hormone that affects sodium and water retention and potassium excretion

6 Outer layer of the adrenal gland

7 Pattern of steroid hormone release

DOWN

1 Steroid hormone that increases blood glucose levels and fat deposits and breaks down protein for energy

2 Inner layer of the adrenal gland

3 Neurotransmitter released from the adrenal medulla

4 Anterior pituitary hormone that causes release of corticosteroids

5 Steroid hormones produced by the adrenal cortex

■ True or False

Indicate whether the following statements are true (T) or false (F).

_____ 1. There are two adrenal glands, one on either side of the kidney.

_____ 2. The adrenal cortex is basically a sympathetic nerve ganglia that releases norepinephrine and epinephrine into the bloodstream in response to sympathetic stimulation.

_____ 3. The adrenal medulla produces three corticosteroids: androgens (male and female sex hormones), glucocorticoids, and mineralocorticoids.

_____ 4. The corticosteroids are released normally in a diurnal rhythm.

_____ 5. Prolonged use of corticosteroids will suppress the normal hypothalamic–pituitary axis and lead to adrenal atrophy from lack of stimulation.

_____ 6. The glucocorticoids decrease glucose production, stimulate fat deposition and protein breakdown, and increase protein formation.

_____ 7. The mineralocorticoids stimulate sodium and water excretion and potassium retention.

_____ 8. Adverse effects of corticosteroids are related to exaggeration of their physiological effects, including immunosuppression, peptic ulcer formation, fluid retention, and edema.

_____ 9. Corticosteroids are used topically and locally to achieve the desired anti-inflammatory effects.

_____ 10. Glucocorticoids are used in conjunction with mineralocorticoids to treat adrenal insufficiency.

■ Patient Teaching Checklist

Stan is an active 16-year-old boy with Crohn's disease. He has been doing quite well until this week when he was admitted with severe inflammation of the large intestine, pain, bloody diarrhea, fever, and dehydration. He is started on prednisone to calm the inflammation while further studies are done to evaluate his disease. Anticipating that Stan will be taking prednisone for at least a few weeks, prepare a patient teaching checklist for him.

CHAPTER 37

Thyroid and Parathyroid Agents

■ Patient Teaching Checklist

P. K. is a 34-year-old mother of three who has been experiencing increasing fatigue, hair loss, apathy, sweating spells, and heart palpitations. After several diagnostic tests, it was discovered that she has hypothyroidism. She was started on levothyroxine, 150 μg/d. Her dose will be adjusted based on her response to the medication. Prepare a drug teaching card for P. K. to take with her when she leaves the office today.

■ Multiple Choice

Select the best answer for the following.

1. Thyroid hormones control:
   a. the rate at which most body cells use energy (metabolism).
   b. release of adrenocorticotropic hormone (ACTH).
   c. the growth of long bones.
   d. ovulation.

2. Control of the thyroid gland involves:
   a. parathyroid hormones.
   b. balanced levels of ACTH.
   c. an intricate balance between the hypothalamus, the anterior pituitary, and circulating levels of thyroid hormone.
   d. a positive feedback system.

3. Hypothyroidism is:
   a. treatable with diet changes.
   b. easily diagnosed in the elderly.
   c. lower-than-normal levels of thyroid hormone.
   d. treated with thioamides.

4. Hyperthyroidism is:
   a. lower-than-normal levels of thyroid hormone.
   b. treatable only with surgical intervention.
   c. treated with radioactive iodine.
   d. treated with thioamides or with iodines.

5. The parathyroid glands:
   a. secrete calcitonin.
   b. are located behind the thyroid gland.

c. are palpable when enlarged.

d. secrete calcium when serum calcium levels are low.

6. Bisphosphonates:

a. raise serum calcium levels.

b. are used to treat hypocalcemia.

c. increase the excretion of sodium from the kidney.

d. slow or block bone resorption.

■ Matching

Match the following words with the appropriate choice.

1. _____ iodine
2. _____ thyroxine
3. _____ liothyronine
4. _____ calcitonin
5. _____ hypothyroidism
6. _____ cretinism
7. _____ myxedema
8. _____ hyperthyroidism
9. _____ thioamides
10. _____ Paget's disease

A. T_4

B. Hormone produced by the thyroid

C. Lack of thyroid hormone in the infant

D. Excess levels of thyroid hormone

E. Dietary element used to produce thyroid hormone

F. T_3

G. Drugs used to prevent the formation of thyroid hormone

H. Severe lack of thyroid hormone in adults

I. Disorder of overactive osteoclasts

J. Lack of sufficient thyroid hormone to maintain metabolism

■ Word Scramble

Unscramble the following letters to form words related to thyroid and parathyroid glands.

1. ccnniiloat _____
2. oxtnihery _____
3. mertiiscn _____
4. sseothapnsoihbp _____
5. thromonearap _____
6. inodei _____
7. oooossstepir _____
8. mhstirdeipoyrhy _____
9. madeyemx _____
10. irioontihnye _____

CHAPTER 38

Antidiabetic Agents

■ Word Search

Circle the following names of antidiabetic agents that are hidden in the following grid.

acarbose
acetohexamide
chlorpropamide
glimepiride
glipizide
glyburide
insulin
metformin
miglitol
repaglinide
sulfonylurea
tolazamide
tolbutamide

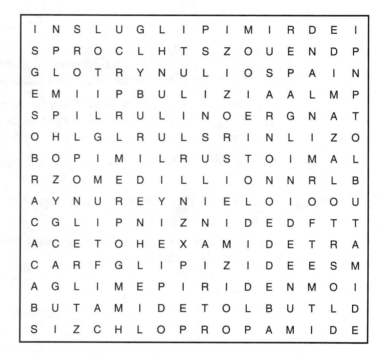

```
I  N  S  L  U  G  L  I  P  I  M  I  R  D  E  I
S  P  R  O  C  L  H  T  S  Z  O  U  E  N  D  P
G  L  O  T  R  Y  N  U  L  I  O  S  P  A  I  N
E  M  I  I  P  B  U  L  I  Z  I  A  A  L  M  P
S  P  I  L  R  U  L  I  N  O  E  R  G  N  A  T
O  H  L  G  L  R  U  L  S  R  I  N  L  I  Z  O
B  O  P  I  M  I  L  R  U  S  T  O  I  M  A  L
R  Z  O  M  E  D  I  L  L  I  O  N  N  R  L  B
A  Y  N  U  R  E  Y  N  I  E  L  O  I  O  O  U
C  G  L  I  P  N  I  Z  N  I  D  E  D  F  T  T
A  C  E  T  O  H  E  X  A  M  I  D  E  T  R  A
C  A  R  F  G  L  I  P  I  Z  I  D  E  E  S  M
A  G  L  I  M  E  P  I  R  I  D  E  N  M  O  I
B  U  T  A  M  I  D  E  T  O  L  B  U  T  L  D
S  I  Z  C  H  L  O  P  R  O  P  A  M  I  D  E
```

■ Web Exercise

J. L. is a 53-year-old traveling salesman recently diagnosed with type 2 diabetes. He and his family are referred to the nurse for education about his disease, diet, drugs, and medical regimen. Go to the Internet to find the latest information for J. L. and to prepare the best teaching resources for him and his family.

■ Nursing Care Plan

P. G. is a 78-year-old post–myocardial infarction patient with diabetes who is admitted to your assisted living facility. He is on propranolol (Inderal) to prevent reinfarction and insulin. Prepare a nursing care plan for his chart to promote continuity of care with his insulin therapy.

■ Fill In The Blanks

1. The most common metabolic disorder in this country is _____ _____ .

2. The pancreas produces three different hormones, all related to glucose control. These three hormones are: _____, _____, and _____ .

3. Insulin stimulates the synthesis of _____ (stored glucose for immediate release during times of stress or low glucose), the conversion of _____ into fat stored in the form of adipose tissue, and the synthesis of needed _____ from amino acids.

4. Hyperglycemia results in _____ as sugar is spilled into the urine.

5. Hyperglycemia will also cause _____ (increased eating) because the hypothalamic centers cannot take in glucose and sense that they are starving.

6. _____ (increased thirst) occurs with hyperglycemia because the tonicity of the blood is increased due to the increased glucose and waste products in the blood and to the loss of fluid with glucose in the urine.

7. When a person with diabetes needs to break down fats for energy, he or she will experience _____ as the metabolism shifts from using sugar to the use of fat and the ketone wastes that result cannot be removed effectively.

8. The first steps for controlling diabetes should always be _____ and _____ .

9. The _____ were the first oral antidiabetic agents. They stimulate the pancreas to produce more insulin.

10. _____ is an oral antidiabetic agent that decreases the production of glucose and increases its uptake into cells.

Introduction to the Reproductive System

■ Fill in the Blanks

Identify the parts of the female reproductive system. Indicate where the ova are stored and the site of estrogen and progesterone production.

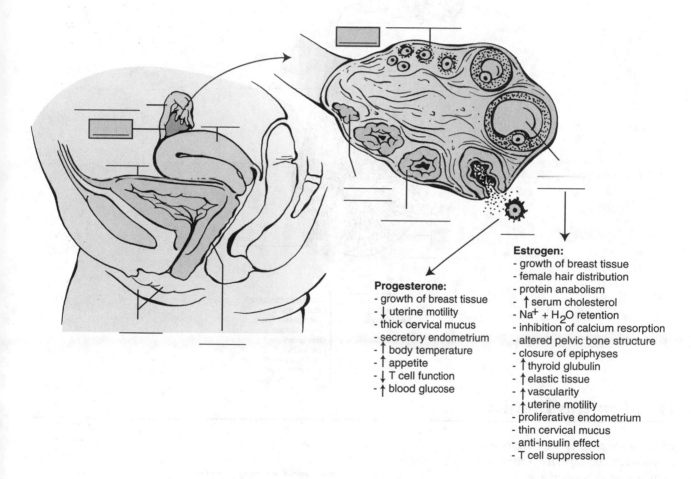

Progesterone:
- growth of breast tissue
- ↓ uterine motility
- thick cervical mucus
- secretory endometrium
- ↑ body temperature
- ↑ appetite
- ↓ T cell function
- ↑ blood glucose

Estrogen:
- growth of breast tissue
- female hair distribution
- protein anabolism
- ↑ serum cholesterol
- Na^+ + H_2O retention
- inhibition of calcium resorption
- altered pelvic bone structure
- closure of epiphyses
- ↑ thyroid glubulin
- ↑ elastic tissue
- ↑ vascularity
- ↑ uterine motility
- proliferative endometrium
- thin cervical mucus
- anti-insulin effect
- T cell suppression

■ Fill in the Blanks

Identify the parts of the male reproductive system. Indicate the site of sperm and testosterone production.

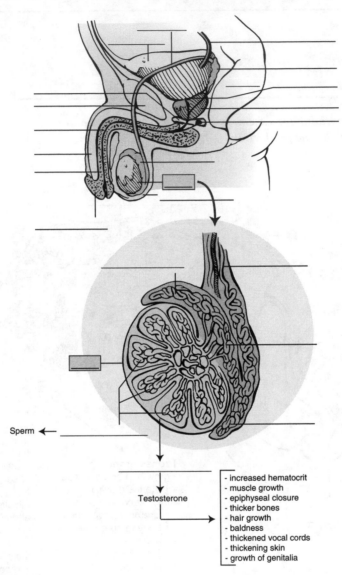

■ Fill in the Blanks

Fill in the names of the hormones involved in the negative feedback system that controls the male reproductive system.

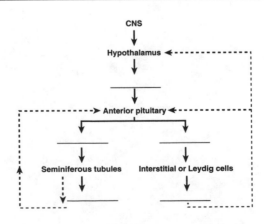

■ Word Search

Circle the following words related to the reproductive system hidden in the following grid. Words may appear diagonally, vertically, or horizontally.

corpus luteum
cycle
estrogen
fallopian
follicle
inhibin
interstitial
Leydig cells
menopause
menstrual
ova
ovaries
ovulation
progesterone
puberty
seminiferous tubules
sperm
testes
testosterone
uterus

A	I	A	A	O	E	E	S	U	S	T	E	H	T	N	T	T	A	H	I	C	O	S	U
N	T	M	L	N	W	D	O	A	G	U	I	G	E	E	H	A	O	K	L	L	E	E	N
H	P	O	O	E	D	O	Z	A	L	A	G	A	T	A	B	U	L	C	Y	L	R	I	T
E	N	N	R	E	C	T	L	A	U	R	T	S	N	E	M	O	M	Y	U	E	H	R	U
C	A	E	I	M	O	E	S	A	A	T	O	M	T	I	R	B	A	B	S	Y	Y	A	R
H	I	G	H	P	R	O	G	E	S	T	E	R	O	N	E	L	U	I	K	D	A	V	S
I	P	O	W	Y	T	C	A	V	N	H	R	E	V	S	P	T	T	A	P	I	I	O	N
C	O	R	P	U	S	L	U	T	E	U	M	P	A	I	S	E	E	L	C	G	A	D	N
W	L	T	H	A	T	E	L	F	I	O	D	U	O	U	Y	S	R	N	A	C	C	E	S
Y	L	S	N	T	E	S	T	O	S	T	E	R	O	N	E	T	U	S	T	E	E	D	F
O	A	E	O	U	R	G	V	R	A	D	E	R	U	R	T	E	S	D	N	L	E	I	R
N	F	E	I	D	L	O	C	Y	C	L	E	A	R	A	N	S	A	N	D	L	S	H	E
R	E	T	T	R	E	I	E	I	S	F	O	L	L	I	C	L	E	U	O	S	Y	E	L
O	F	Y	A	O	Y	R	C	O	I	N	T	E	R	S	T	I	T	I	A	L	C	E	L
R	S	E	L	E	T	U	I	N	H	I	B	I	N	T	E	N	O	L	A	S	E	V	A
M	T	H	U	I	A	M	I	S	O	V	E	P	U	B	E	R	T	Y	R	Y	L	O	N
O	N	S	V	Y	M	M	E	N	O	P	A	U	S	E	D	I	S	Y	I	M	Y	L	E
U	I	C	O	P	E	C	E	I	T	R	A	D	A	N	Y	E	C	W	M	U	O	Y	S
S	O	E	R	S	E	A	P	N	S	E	N	W	O	P	R	I	E	E	B	E	H	A	P

CHAPTER 40

Drugs Affecting the Female Reproductive System

■ Crossword Puzzle

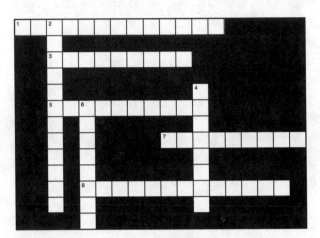

ACROSS

1 Drug used to stimulate evacuation of the uterus
3 Uterine relaxant
5 Female sex hormones, important in maintaining a pregnancy
7 Type of drugs used to stimulate ovulation and pregnancy
8 Birth control measure

DOWN

2 Loss of calcium from the bone
4 Primary female sex hormone
6 Drug that stimulates uterine contraction and milk ejection

■ Multiple Choice

Select the best answer to the following.

1. Estrogens are **not**:
   a. female sex hormones important in the development of the female reproductive system and secondary sex characteristics.
   b. used pharmacologically mainly to replace hormones lost at menopause.
   c. used to stimulate ovulation in woman with hypogonadism.
   d. used to treat uterine bleeding problems.

2. Progestins:
   a. are used in combination with estrogens for oral contraceptives.
   b. are not necessary during pregnancy and lactation.
   c. are responsible for a thin, clear cervical mucous.
   d. cause growth of long bones at puberty.

3. Fertility drugs:
   a. can stimulate ovulation in postmenopausal women.
   b. have a major adverse effect of multiple births and birth defects.
   c. directly stimulate gonadotropin-releasing hormone (GnRH) release from the hypothalamus.
   d. are not associated with adverse effects unless pregnancy occurs.

4. Oxytocic drugs:
   a. can act as fertility drugs because they stimulate the hypothalamus.
   b. stimulate uterine contractions and induce or speed up labor.
   c. cannot be used postpartum.
   d. are like the posterior pituitary hormone antidiuretic hormone (ADH).

5. Abortifacients:
   a. can be used through the third trimester of pregnancy.
   b. are drugs that stimulate uterine activity to cause uterine evacuation.
   c. can be used to induce labor at term.
   d. are not associated with any adverse effects.

6. Tocolytics:
   a. stimulate uterine contractions.
   b. are good fertility drugs.
   c. relax the uterine smooth muscle to stop premature labor.
   d. can be used as contraceptives.

■ Word Scramble

Unscramble the following letters to form the names of commonly used estrogens and estrogen receptor modulators.

1. morefinete _____
2. dotrailse _____
3. noreest _____
4. foxnarliee _____
5. notsiederl _____
6. potrestapei _____
7. stillbesthiedyrotl _____
8. cehnleosriontari _____

■ Fill in the Blanks

1. Drugs that stimulate uterine contractions are called _____.

2. Drugs that are used to relax the gravid uterus to prolong pregnancy are referred to as _____.

3. Loss of estrogen is associated with many problems at menopause, including _____ or a loss of calcium from the bones, _____ _____ associated with vascular spasms, and an increased risk of _____ _____ _____, the leading cause of death among women.

4. Women are strongly discouraged from smoking when taking estrogen replacement therapy because of an increased risk of _____ and _____ development.

5. _____ is an estrogen receptor modulator, stimulating some receptors and blocking others.

6. Levonorgestrel, a _____, is available in the form of an implanted contraceptive system.

7. Women without primary ovarian failure who cannot become pregnant after a year of trying may be candidates for the use of _____.

8. Drugs that can be used to induce abortion in early pregnancy or to promote uterine evacuation after intrauterine fetal death are called _____.

CHAPTER 41

Drugs Affecting the Male Reproductive System

■ True or False

Indicate whether the following statements are true (T) or false (F).

_____ 1. Androgens are male sex hormones, specifically testosterone or testosterone-like compounds.

_____ 2. Androgens are responsible for the development and maintenance of male sex characteristics and secondary sex characteristics or estrogenic effects.

_____ 3. Adverse effects related to androgen use involve potentially deadly hepatocellular carcinoma.

_____ 4. Androgens can be used for replacement therapy or to block other hormone effects.

_____ 5. Anabolic steroids are analogs of estrogen that have been developed to have protein building effects.

_____ 6. Anabolic steroids are used pharmacologically to enhance muscle development and athletic performance, often with deadly effects.

_____ 7. Anabolic steroids are used to increase hematocrit and improve protein anabolism in certain depleted states.

_____ 8. Erectile penile dysfunction can inhibit erection and male sexual function.

_____ 9. Alprostadil, a prostaglandin, is an oral agent used to stimulate penile erection.

_____ 10. Sildenafil is an injected agent that acts quickly to promote vascular filling of the corpus cavernosum and promote penile erection.

■ Matching

Match the drug with its usual indication.

1. _____ nandrolone
2. _____ oxandrolone
3. _____ oxymetholone
4. _____ stanozolol
5. _____ danazol
6. _____ fluoxymesterone
7. _____ testolactone
8. _____ testosterone

A. Treatment of anemias

B. Treatment of specific breast cancers

C. Blocks follicle-stimulating hormone (FSH) and luteinizing hormone (LH) release in women

D. Anemia associated with renal dysfunction

E. Promotion of weight gain

F. Primary male sex hormone—treatment of hypogonadism and certain breast cancers

G. Treatment of angioedema

H. Replacement therapy in hypogonadism

■ Fill in the Blanks

1. _____ effects are associated with development of male sexual characteristics.

2. _____ effects are tissue-building effects associated with androgen use.

3. _____ is the primary natural androgen.

4. Because they cause an increase in red blood cell production, androgens may be indicated to treat various _____.

5. _____ is a condition in which the corpus cavernosum does not fill with blood to allow for penile erection.

6. Alprostadil is a _____ that relaxes vascular smooth muscle and allows filling of the corpus cavernosum when _____ directly into the cavernosum.

7. _____ is taken orally and acts to increase nitrous oxide levels in the corpus cavernosum.

8. The penile erection that accompanies oral use of *Viagra* occurs only with _____.

■ Word Scramble

Unscramble the following letters to form words related to the drugs affecting the male reproductive system.

1. ssiihurtm _____

2. pydmishnogoa _____

3. bolainca _____

4. asfilldne _____

5. gorednnsa _____

6. eeertcli cydtsifuonn _____

7. ttteeessoonr _____

8. palsordatli _____

9. droneloann _____

10. zoandla _____

CHAPTER 42

Introduction to the Cardiovascular System

■ Fill in the Blanks

Fill in the blanks indicating the structures in the heart.

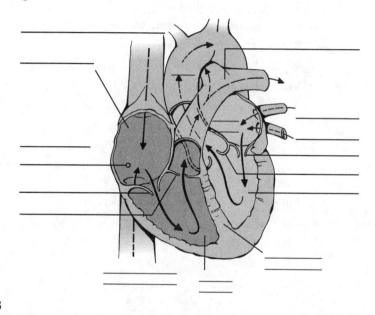

■ Definitions

Define the following terms.

1. troponin _____
   _____

2. actin _____
   _____

3. myosin _____
   _____

4. arrhythmia _____
   _____

5. Starling's law of the heart _____
   _____

6. fibrillation _____
   _____

7. capillary _____

_____

8. resistance system _____

_____

■ Matching

Match the word with the appropriate definition.

1. _____ atrium
2. _____ ventricle
3. _____ auricle
4. _____ vein
5. _____ artery
6. _____ myocardium
7. _____ syncytia
8. _____ diastole
9. _____ systole
10. _____ automaticity
11. _____ conductivity
12. _____ pulse pressure

A. Resting phase of the heart
B. Reflects the filling pressure of the coronary arteries
C. Bottom chamber of the heart
D. Vessel that takes blood away from the heart
E. Vessel that returns blood to the heart
F. Appendage on the atria of the heart
G. Property of heart cells to generate an action potential
H. Top chamber of the heart
I. Property of heart cells to rapidly conduct an action potential of electrical impulse
J. Intertwining network of muscle fibers
K. Contracting phase of the heart
L. Muscle of the heart

■ Crossword Puzzle

Fill in the following spaces with words from the word list that relate to the cardiovascular system.

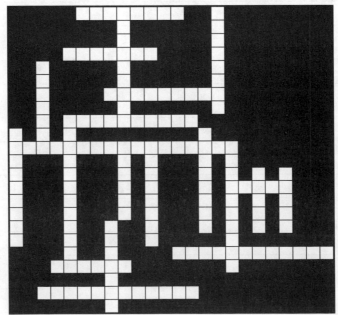

ACTIN
CYCLE
VEINS
ATRIUM
MYOSIN
AURICLE
CARDIAC
SYSTOLE
ARTERIES
DIASTOLE
SYNCYTIA
TROPONIN
CAPILLARY
SARCOMERE
VENTRICLE
ARRHYTHMIA
MYOCARDIUM
AUTOMATICITY
CONDUCTIVITY
FIBRILLATION
ELECTROCARDIOGRAM

CHAPTER 43

Drugs Affecting Blood Pressure

■ Matching

Match the following drugs with their appropriate class of antihypertensive agents.
(Some classes may be used more than once.)

1. _____ candesartan

2. _____ quinapril

3. _____ mecamylamine

4. _____ losartan

5. _____ nitroprusside

6. _____ tolazoline

7. _____ lisinopril

8. _____ valsartan

9. _____ nicardipine

10. _____ minoxidil

11. _____ fosinopril

12. _____ amlodipine

A. Angiotensin-converting enzyme inhibitor
B. Angiotensin II receptor blocker
C. Calcium channel blocker
D. Vasodilator
E. Ganglionic blocker

■ Word Search

Circle the following names of antihypertensive agents that are hidden in the following grid.

benazepril
candesartan
diazoxide
captopril
losartan
minoxidil
enalapril
valsartan
nitroprusside
ramipril
amlodipine
mecamylamine
trandolapril
diltiazem
nicardipine

M	I	N	O	X	I	D	I	P	I	N	E	N	A	L
P	E	R	L	I	R	P	A	L	A	N	E	I	L	E
B	R	A	M	L	O	D	I	P	I	N	E	I	V	E
S	N	I	C	A	R	D	I	P	I	N	E	T	A	L
D	I	A	Z	E	P	U	L	M	D	E	D	R	L	L
I	N	A	L	A	P	R	A	B	I	D	I	A	S	I
L	O	R	S	A	R	L	I	S	I	B	S	N	A	R
T	O	R	A	V	Y	A	Z	I	D	E	S	D	R	P
I	N	A	L	M	E	T	R	O	P	L	U	O	T	O
A	E	W	A	O	I	R	I	U	I	E	R	L	A	T
Z	E	C	H	I	P	P	N	O	L	S	P	A	N	P
E	E	S	L	O	S	A	R	T	A	N	O	P	O	A
M	E	D	I	A	Z	O	X	I	D	E	R	R	N	C
B	E	N	A	Z	E	P	R	I	L	T	T	I	E	A
R	L	I	O	M	I	N	O	X	I	D	I	L	L	N
O	C	A	N	D	E	S	A	R	T	A	N	E	L	D

■ True or False

Indicate whether the following statements are true (T) or false (F).

_____ 1. The cardiovascular system is an open system that depends on pressure differences to ensure the delivery of blood.

_____ 2. Blood pressure is related to heart rate, stroke volume, and the total peripheral resistance.

_____ 3. Constricted arterioles lower pressure; dilated arterioles raise pressure.

_____ 4. Control of blood pressure involves baroreceptor (pressure receptor) stimulation of the medulla to activate the parasympathetic nervous system.

_____ 5. The kidneys activate the renin-angiotensin system when blood flow to the kidneys is decreased.

_____ 6. Renin activates angiotensinogen to angiotensin I in the lung using angiotensin-converting enzyme.

_____ 7. Hypertension is a sustained state of higher-than-normal blood pressure.

_____ 8. Essential hypertension has no underlying cause, and treatment can vary widely.

_____ 9. Angiotensin II receptor blockers prevent the body from responding to angiotensin II and blocking calcium channels.

_____ 10. Hypotension can result in decreased oxygenation of the tissues, cell death, tissue damage, and even death.

■ Matching

Match the antihypertensive agent with the commonly used brand name.

1. _____ benazepril
2. _____ hydralazine
3. _____ candesartan
4. _____ quinapril
5. _____ diltiazem
6. _____ losartan
7. _____ captopril
8. _____ nifedipine
9. _____ lisinopril
10. _____ moexipril

A. *Cozaar*
B. *Univasc*
C. *Accupril*
D. *Lotensin*
E. *Procardia XL*
F. *Atacand*
G. *Capoten*
H. *Zestril*
I. *Apresoline*
J. *Cardizem*

CHAPTER 44

Cardiotonic Agents

■ Patient Teaching Checklist

F. A. is a 72-year-old woman with mitral valve disease. She has been doing fairly well until this summer, when she went into congestive heart failure (CHF). She has been stabilized on digoxin (Lanoxin). She moves to Florida every November for 6 months. Prepare a teaching card for her to take with her to ensure continuity of care when she switches to her Florida health care provider.

■ Crossword Puzzle

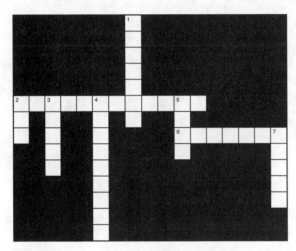

ACROSS

2 Enlargement of the heart
6 Lack of energy

DOWN

1 Difficulty breathing
2 Congestive heart failure

3 Side of the heart associated with total body congestion
4 Difficulty breathing while lying down
5 Side of the heart associated with pulmonary edema
7 Swelling

■ Web Exercise

J. D. calls your clinic asking for information about CHF. Her mother has been diagnosed with CHF, and J. D. is moving her to town so that she can care for her. However, J. D. does not know anything about CHF and wants to find out what she can expect. Use the Internet to obtain information that might be useful to J. D.

■ Word Scramble

Unscramble the following letters to form words related to the cardiotonic agents.

1. pnseyad _____

2. oneiirnlm _____

3. catoniur _____

4. topranheo _____

5. haptaceny _____

6. voteginsec thrae firaleu _____

7. nixgodi _____

8. potymsehis _____

9. yohitdarpaocmy _____

10. unimem abf _____

CHAPTER 45

Antiarrhythmic Agents

■ Fill in the Blanks

Identify the parts of the cardiac conduction system.

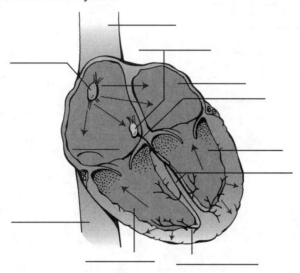

■ Matching

Match the following arrhythmia with the name of the arrhythmia and a drug commonly used to treat it.

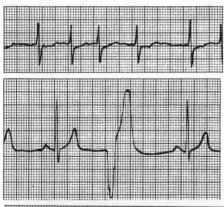

A. Premature ventricular contractions (PVC)
B. Atrial fibrillation
C. Ventricular flutter
D. Quinidine
E. Amiodarone
F. Lidocaine

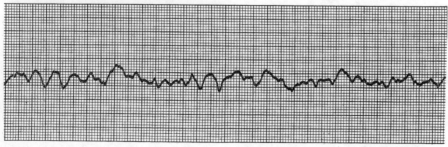

■ Word Scramble

Unscramble the following letters to form the names of commonly used antiarrhythmic agents.

1. namedooria _____

2. moolesl _____

3. bytermiul _____

4. apevirmal _____

5. moperacnidia _____

6. pdolproran _____

7. inifledeca _____

8. onidigx _____

■ Fill In The Blanks

1. Arrhythmias can be caused by changes in heart rate, either _____ or _____.

2. Arrhythmias can cause a decrease in _____, leading to a decrease in the blood being pumped to the brain and periphery.

3. Antiarrhythmics alter the _____ of the heart cells and interfere with conduction, blocking arrhythmias.

4. Long-term treatment of arrhythmias is no longer considered prudent because of the results of the _____ _____.

5. Cardiac cells possess the property of _____, allowing them to generate an action potential but also making them susceptible to arrhythmias.

6. Class II antiarrhythmics are _____ _____ blockers

7. A drug that is a commonly used cardiotonic agent that is used to slow the heart rate and treat atrial arrhythmias is _____.

8. _____ is frequently used to treat ventricular arrhythmias in emergency situations and is also a commonly used local anesthetic.

CHAPTER 46

Antianginal Agents

■ Matching

Match the word with the appropriate definition.

1. _____ CAD
2. _____ pulse pressure
3. _____ atheroma
4. _____ atherosclerosis
5. _____ angina pectoris
6. _____ Prinzmetal's angina
7. _____ myocardial infarction
8. _____ nitrates

A. "Suffocation of the chest"

B. Drop in blood flow through the coronary arteries caused by a vasospasm in the artery

C. Coronary artery disease

D. End result of vessel blockage in the heart

E. Fatty tumor in the intima of a coronary artery

F. Filling pressure of the coronary arteries

G. Narrowing of the arteries caused by buildup of atheromas

H. Drugs used to cause direct relaxation of smooth muscle

■ True or False

Indicate whether the following statements are true (T) or false (F).

_____ 1. Coronary artery disease (CAD) is second to cancer as the leading cause of death in the United States and most Western nations.

_____ 2. CAD develops when changes in the intima of coronary vessels lead to the development of atheromas, or fatty tumors.

_____ 3. Narrowing of the coronary arteries secondary to the atheroma buildup is called angina.

_____ 4. Angina pectoris, or "suffocation of the chest," occurs when the narrowed vessels cannot meet the myocardial demand for oxygen.

_____ 5. Stable angina occurs when the heart muscle is perfused adequately except at rest.

_____ 6. Unstable or preinfarction angina occurs when the vessels are so narrowed that the myocardial cells are low on oxygen during exertion.

_____ 7. Prinzmetal's angina occurs as a result of a spasm of a coronary vessel.

_____ 8. Myocardial infarction occurs when a coronary vessel is completely occluded.

■ Crossword Puzzle

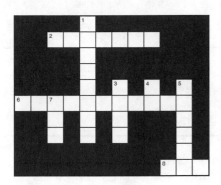

ACROSS

2 Vasodilator
6 Lack of oxygen
8 Leading cause of death in U.S.

4 Myocardial infarction
5 Suffocation of the chest
7 Component of an atheroma

DOWN

1 Fatty tumor in the lumen of a vessel
3 Symptom of angina

■ Word Search

Circle the following words related to angina and antianginal drugs hidden in the following grid. Words may appear diagonally, vertically, or horizontally.

angina
atheroma
atherosclerosis
CAD
myocardial infarction
calcium channel
coronary artery
diltiazem
exertion
metoprolol
nitrates
nitroglycerin
pain
pectoris
pressure
Prinzmetal's
propranolol
pulse
pulse pressure
verapamil

U	E	R	E	K	R	E	E	R	U	S	S	E	R	P	E	L	D	D	S	M	H
S	D	N	V	E	R	A	P	A	M	I	L	T	H	R	U	E	I	T	I	W	T
N	A	I	O	U	A	T	H	E	R	O	M	A	U	I	R	L	H	R	R	E	T
L	C	T	W	T	N	T	R	P	A	I	N	S	G	N	E	N	S	A	R	N	A
C	F	R	G	O	G	T	H	A	G	Y	S	O	I	Z	D	A	R	E	O	I	M
D	O	A	S	K	I	E	D	E	R	E	M	F	L	M	I	M	U	N	E	R	N
Y	L	T	I	N	N	O	T	I	R	L	E	H	T	E	C	E	M	O	K	E	C
M	O	E	R	E	A	L	E	P	A	O	D	I	L	T	I	A	Z	E	M	C	I
E	L	S	O	E	L	O	E	R	M	F	S	R	A	A	L	O	G	X	C	Y	H
A	O	H	T	W	H	S	B	E	R	E	S	C	S	L	N	E	D	E	C	L	B
A	R	D	C	E	L	S	O	R	E	P	Y	E	L	S	T	E	R	R	A	G	B
A	P	L	E	U	T	R	K	I	H	A	N	I	P	E	E	I	R	T	B	O	B
V	O	R	P	R	O	P	R	A	N	O	L	O	L	D	R	E	V	I	C	R	O
A	T	R	E	P	S	E	A	C	C	E	S	P	U	P	A	O	R	O	H	T	N
E	E	I	Y	R	E	T	R	A	Y	R	A	N	O	R	O	C	S	N	T	I	O
D	M	Y	O	C	A	R	D	I	A	L	I	N	F	A	R	C	T	I	O	N	N
E	C	A	L	C	I	U	M	C	H	A	N	N	E	L	D	A	S	E	S	A	O
H	T	O	W	H	I	N	L	E	H	L	E	B	R	O	C	L	A	O	T	T	P

Lipid-Lowering Agents

■ Web Exercise

R. K. is a 46-year-old man who is diagnosed with hypertension and elevated low-density lipoproteins (LDLs) during a routine insurance physical. He has a strong family history of heart disease and is concerned about the findings. He is referred to the nurse for appropriate teaching. Use the Internet to obtain the most recent information that might be useful for R. K., then prepare a teaching program for him.

■ Listing

List the leading risk factors for the development of coronary artery disease. Indicate the ones that are modifiable with an M.

1. _____
2. _____
3. _____
4. _____
5. _____
6. _____
7. _____
8. _____
9. _____
10. _____

■ Fill in the Blanks

Identify the process of fat metabolism in humans by filling in the blanks in the following figure. Indicate the site of action of the major classes of lipid-lowering agents.

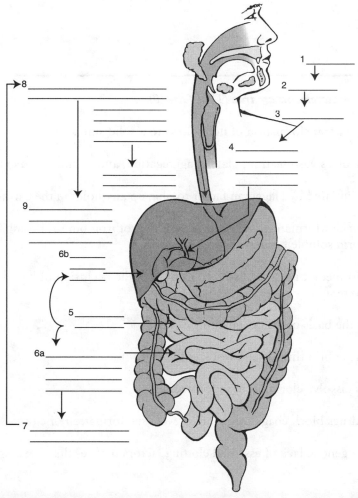

■ Word Scramble

Unscramble the following letters to form words related to lipid-lowering therapy.

1. leolroehtcs _____
2. boretaclif _____
3. nniica _____
4. hypipdeermliia _____
5. cpoolleits _____
6. vastraottina _____
7. fizemiglrob _____
8. lebi scaid _____
9. ppooiilntre _____
10. statviolna _____

Drugs Affecting Blood Coagulation

■ True or False

Indicate whether the following statements are true (T) or false (F).

_____ 1. Coagulation is the transformation of fluid blood to a solid state.

_____ 2. Coagulation involves vasodilation, platelet aggregation, and intrinsic and extrinsic clot formation.

_____ 3. Coagulation is initiated by Hageman factor to plug up any holes in the cardiovascular system.

_____ 4. The final step of clot formation is the conversion of prothrombin to thrombin, which breaks down fibrinogen to form soluble fibrin threads.

_____ 5. Once a clot is formed, it must be dissolved to prevent the occlusion of blood vessels and loss of blood supply to tissues.

_____ 6. Plasminogen is the basis of the coagulation system.

_____ 7. Plasmin dissolves fibrin threads and resolves the clot.

_____ 8. Anticoagulants dissolve clots that have formed.

_____ 9. Thrombolytic drugs block coagulation and prevent the formation of clots.

_____ 10. Hemophilia is a genetic lack of essential clotting factors that results in excessive bleeding situations.

■ Fill in the Blanks

Fill in the blanks in the following figure to identify the steps in the coagulation process.

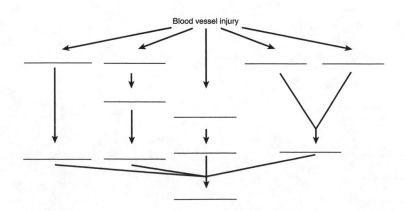

■ Patient Teaching Checklist

C. F. is a 36-year-old mother of three who has recently undergone a mitral valve replacement. She is being stabilized on Coumadin *to prevent the formation of clots as a result of the valve. Prepare a drug teaching card for C. F. that she can refer to at home.*

■ Crossword Puzzle

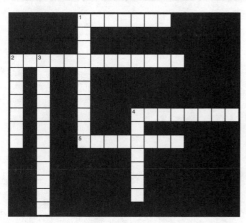

ACROSS

1 Anticoagulant that prevents the conversion of prothrombin to thrombin
2 Prevents clotting
4 Cellular blood component that plugs small holes in blood vessels
5 Anticoagulant that blocks the production of clotting factors

DOWN

1 Stops blood loss
2 Platelet inhibitor used to reduce clot formation
3 Breaks apart blood clots
4 Blood protein that lyses blood clots

CHAPTER 49

Drugs Used to Treat Anemias

■ Fill in the Blanks

Fill in the following blanks to identify the steps of erythropoiesis.

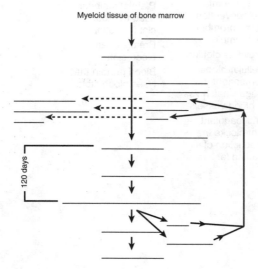

Myeloid tissue of bone marrow

120 days

■ Multiple Choice

Select the best answer to the following.

1. Blood is composed of:
   a. a liquid plasma (containing water, proteins, glucose, and electrolytes).
   b. formed components, including nitrogen and urea.
   c. endothelial cells.
   d. alveolar cells.

2. Erythropoiesis is controlled by:
   a. iron formation.
   b. carbohydrate availability.
   c. erythropoietin, which is produced by the kidneys.
   d. bilirubin.

3. Red blood cells (RBCs):
   a. have a nucleus.
   b. have a life span of about 120 days.
   c. are mostly bilirubin.
   d. have many different shapes.

4. Anemia cannot be caused by:
   a. a lack of erythropoietin.
   b. a lack of the components needed to produce RBCs.
   c. a depressed bone marrow.
   d. increased RBC production.

5. Iron deficiency anemia occurs:
   a. when there is inadequate iron intake in the diet.
   b. when too much iron is absorbed from the gastrointestinal (GI) tract.
   c. when oxygen levels are very low.
   d. when bilirubin is unconjugated.

6. Pernicious anemia is:
   a. a lack of folic acid.
   b. a lack of iron.
   c. a lack of vitamin B_{12}.
   d. not a life-threatening condition.

■ Crossword Puzzle

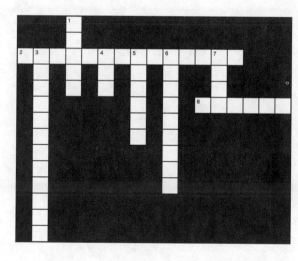

ACROSS

2 Hormone that controls RBC production
8 Lack of RBCs

DOWN

1 Main constituent of plasma
3 Immature RBC
4 Red blood cell
5 Liquid part of the blood
6 Factor that activates folic acid
7 Component of the RBC that allows the cell to carry oxygen

■ Word Scramble

Unscramble the following letters to form words related to anemias.

1. tryhertyesco _____

2. laamsp _____

3. gamelasticbo _____

4. sinpicroue _____

5. tipnoee _____

6. cloif dica _____

7. maneai _____

8. eproyitehsrios _____

9. coryetteucil _____

10. fineccediy _____

CHAPTER 50

Introduction to the Kidney and the Urinary Tract

■ Fill in the Blanks

Fill in the blanks in the following figure to identify the parts of the nephron.

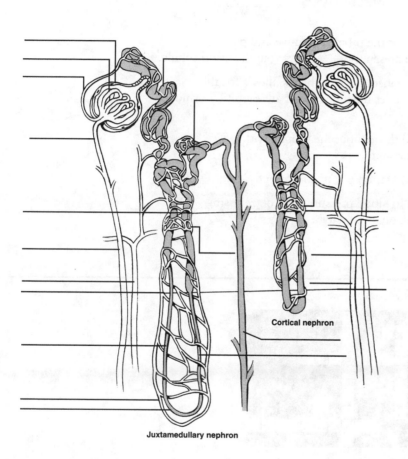

Cortical nephron

Juxtamedullary nephron

■ Word Scramble

Unscramble the following letters to form words associated with the renal system.

1. rumsoulgel _____

2. nattrofili _____

3. tonisceer _____

4. enrootladse _____

5. proberostani _____

6. ubluetu _____

7. niner _____

8. streatpo _____

■ Fill in the Blanks

1. The kidneys are two small organs that receive approximately _____ of the cardiac output.

2. The functional unit of the kidney is called the _____, which is composed of _____, the proximal convoluted tubule, _____, the distal convoluted tubule, and the _____.

3. The nephrons function by using three basic processes: _____, _____, and _____.

4. Sodium levels are regulated throughout the tubule by active and passive movement and are fine-tuned by the presence of _____ in the distal tubule.

5. The countercurrent mechanism in the medullary nephrons allows for the _____ or _____ of urine under the influence of antidiuretic hormone (ADH) secreted by the hypothalamus.

6. Potassium concentration is regulated throughout the tubule, with _____ being the strongest influence for potassium loss.

7. The kidneys play a key role in the regulation of calcium by activating _____.

8. The kidneys have an important role in blood pressure control, releasing _____ to activate the renin–angiotensin system.

■ Crossword Puzzle

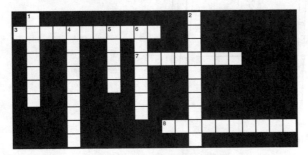

ACROSS

3 Adrenal hormone that regulates K levels
7 Gland
8 Tuft of blood vessel within Bowman's capsule

DOWN

1 Storage site for urinary waiting for excretion
2 Passing through a semipermeable membrane
4 Movement into the tubule
5 Enzyme produced in the JG cells
6 Functional unit of the kidney

CHAPTER 51

Diuretic Agents

■ Word Search

Circle the commonly used diuretics that are hidden in the following grid.

bendroflumethiazide
hydrochlorothiazide
indapamide
trichlormethiazide
metolazone
bumetanide
furosemide
torsemide
acetazolamide
amiloride
spironolactone
glycerin
urea

```
B I D E Z O N E T H I A Z I Z O N E Y L
E H A M I N U R T I Z I D E K L I N D A
N I Y G L Y A T H U A I Z I D E O T O M
D Z E D O E H H I L S O E N O E P R M I
R A C A R B O S T H I A D I D E Z O S T
O I F U R O S E M I D E I I O D R I P S
F H U R O S C M I Z I D M E L I S M I N
L T H E I A Z H I A Z A E L O Z N E R T
U E I D E R O I L Z L Z S I N A D R O S
M M N I R G H I O O I I R N O I R I N T
E U E R O L O O Z L R N O I N H O Z O E
T L F O R Y U A S E M O T A I T D O L E
H F U L R C T F U I A Z T I D E G H A C
I O N I L E H I T L M E H H I F R H C H
A R O M C R U N I M M I O Z I O B E T H
Z D R A I I N U R U N E O S M A T I O I
I N E N L N O R B E M E T O L A Z O N E
D E D I M A P A D N I N E Z I D E I E L
E B T R I C H L O R M E T H I A Z I D E
B Y R O L H I O M O E L H I A Z D E I E
```

■ Definitions

Define the following terms.

1. edema _____

   _____

2. fluid rebound _____

   _____

3. thiazide diuretic _____

_____

4. hypokalemia _____

_____

5. high ceiling diuretics _____

_____

6. alkalosis _____

_____

7. hyperaldosteronism _____

_____

8. osmotic pull _____

_____

■ Matching

Match the diuretic with the appropriate class. (Some classes will be used more than once.)

1. _____ glycerin
2. _____ acetazolamide
3. _____ furosemide
4. _____ benzthiazide
5. _____ indapamide
6. _____ mannitol
7. _____ spironolactone
8. _____ hydrochlorothiazide
9. _____ amiloride
10. _____ bumetanide

A. Osmotic
B. Thiazide
C. Loop
D. Potassium sparing
E. Carbonic anhydrase inhibitor

■ Multiple Choice

Select the best answer to the following.

1. The thiazide diuretics belong to a class of drugs called:
   a. sulfonylureas.
   b. hydroxyureas.
   c. sulfonamides.
   d. sulfa drugs.

2. Thiazide diuretics act in the renal tubule to block the:
   a. potassium pump.
   b. calcium channels.
   c. sodium pump.
   d. chloride pump.

3. One of the common adverse effects associated with most diuretic therapy is:
   a. hyperkalemia.
   b. hypokalemia.
   c. hypocalcemia.
   d. hypercalcemia.

4. Loop diuretics are also called:
   a. thiazide diuretics.
   b. osmotic diuretics.
   c. potassium-sparing diuretics.
   d. high-ceiling diuretics.

5. Carbonic anhydrase inhibitors are diuretics most often used to treat:
   a. glaucoma.
   b. congestive heart failure.
   c. liver failure.
   d. renal failure.

6. Patients who routinely take diuretics should be advised to:
   a. limit their fluid intake as much as possible.
   b. avoid any sodium intake.
   c. always take the drug on an empty stomach.
   d. take the drug early in the day.

7. Patients who would be at risk if their potassium levels fall are often given a potassium-sparing diuretic such as:
   a. furosemide.
   b. spironolactone.
   c. mannitol.
   d. hydrochlorothiazide.

8. Hydrochlorothiazide is commonly found in combination products used to treat:
   a. cirrhosis.
   b. renal failure.
   c. hypertension.
   d. hypotension.

CHAPTER 52

Drugs Affecting the Urinary Tract and Bladder

■ Web Exercise

H. H. and his wife are referred to you for teaching after a diagnosis of benign prostatic hyperplasia (BPH) is made on a routine physical. They do not understand the problem and are somewhat shy talking about it. Go to the Internet to get information for them about the disease, treatment, and research.

■ Patient Teaching Checklist

J. W., a 14-year-old with chronic cystitis, has recently moved from a small town and is seen for the first time at your clinic. She has an active cystitis and is started on cinoxacin. Prepare a teaching checklist for J. W. that includes information regarding prevention of urinary tract infections.

■ True or False

Indicate whether the following statements are true (T) or false (F).

_____ 1. Acute urinary tract infections are second in frequency to respiratory tract infections in the American population.

_____ 2. Urinary tract anti-infectives are used to kill bacteria in the urinary tract by producing alkaline urine or by destroying bacteria in the urinary tract.

_____ 3. There is nothing that can be done to help decrease the bacteria in the urinary tract.

_____ 4. Inflammation and irritation of the urinary tract can cause smooth muscle spasms leading to the uncomfortable effects of dysuria, urgency, incontinence, nocturia, and suprapubic pain.

_____ 5. The urinary tract antispasmodics relieve spasms of the urinary tract muscles by blocking sympathetic activity.

_____ 6. Pentosan polysulfate sodium is a heparin-like compound that has anticoagulant and fibrinolytic effects and is used specifically to decrease the pain and discomfort associated with interstitial cystitis.

_____ 7. BPH is a rare condition that involves enlargement of the prostate gland in older males.

_____ 8. Drugs commonly used to relieve the signs and symptoms of prostate enlargement include α-adrenergic blockers, which relax the sympathetic effects on the bladder and sphincters, and finasteride, which blocks the body's production of a powerful androgen.

■ Word Scramble

Unscramble the following letters to form terms associated with the urinary tract.

1. rayisud _____
2. rantucio _____
3. gunrecy _____
4. eequcnyrf _____
5. iittsscy _____
6. oxazosnid _____
7. nnyyboxuti _____
8. ntcfdcaiiiioa _____
9. pastmansidisco _____
10. onehetpplryiis _____

CHAPTER 53

Introduction to the Respiratory System

■ Fill in the Blanks

Label the parts of the respiratory system in the following figure.

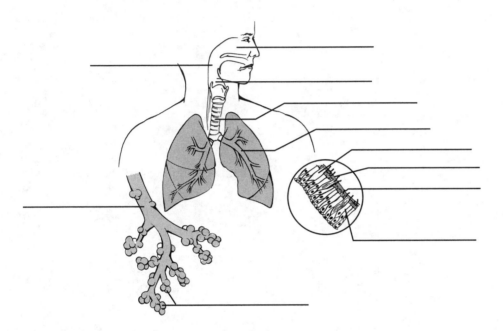

■ Matching

Match the word with the appropriate definition.

1. _____ upper respiratory tract

2. _____ bronchial tree

3. _____ lower respiratory tract

4. _____ alveoli

5. _____ cilia

6. _____ sinuses

7. _____ larynx

8. _____ trachea

9. _____ cough

10. _____ ventilation

11. _____ respiratory membrane

12. _____ surfactant

A. Air-filled passages through the skull

B. The area where gas exchange takes place

C. The vocal chords and the epiglottis

D. The conducting airways leading into the alveoli

E. Microscopic hair-like projections of the epithelial cell membrane

F. The exchange of gases at the alveolar level

G. The main conducting airway leading into the lungs

H. Lipoprotein that reduces surface tension in the alveoli

I. The surface through which gas exchange must occur

J. The respiratory sacs

K. The nose, mouth, pharynx, larynx, trachea, and upper bronchial tree area through which gas exchange must be made

L. Reflex response in the respiratory membrane; results in forced air expelled through the mouth

■ Multiple Choice

Select the best answer to the following.

1. A sneeze:
   a. is a reflex response to irritation in the nasal passages.
   b. results in forced air expelled through the mouth.
   c. involves tight closure of the larynx.
   d. involves sequential contraction of muscles in the esophagus.

2. Ventilation is:
   a. the delivery of blood to the tissues.
   b. the movement of air into the nares.
   c. the exchange of gases at the alveolar-level respiratory membrane.
   d. not affected by changes in the respiratory membrane.

3. The respiratory membrane is composed of:
   a. the capillary cell, the alveolar cell, and the surfactant layer.
   b. the capillary cell, the capillary basement membrane, a fluid layer, a thickened basement membrane, and the alveolar cell.
   c. the capillary basement membrane, the adventitia, the pleura, the alveolar cell, and the surfactant layer.
   d. the capillary cell, the capillary basement membrane, the interstitial space, the alveolar basement membrane, the alveolar cell, and the surfactant layer.

4. The common cold:
   a. blocks the inflammatory response.
   b. prevents the release of histamine and prostaglandins, resulting in a stuffy feeling.
   c. is a viral infection of the upper respiratory tract.
   d. is caused by not wearing a hat in the winter.

5. Seasonal rhinitis is:
   a. another name for the common cold.
   b. caused by a common virus.
   c. caused by an autoimmune reaction.
   d. caused by a reaction to a specific antigen.

6. Pneumonia is:
   a. an inflammation of the epithelial lining of the nasal sinuses.
   b. an inflammation of the lungs.
   c. an inherited deficiency.
   d. usually caused by a reaction to a specific antigen.

7. Asthma:
   a. is a disorder characterized by recurrent episodes of bronchospasm.
   b. is a chronic, never an acute, reaction.
   c. results from repeated attacks of chronic obstructive pulmonary disorder (COPD).
   d. leads to collapse of the alveoli.

8. COPD:

   a. is an acute bronchospasm.

   b. is a chronic condition that occurs over time.

   c. does not alter the physical structure of the lungs.

   d. affects only the very young.

■ Word Search

Circle the words related to the respiratory tract hidden in the following grid. The words may appear diagonally, vertically, or horizontally.

alveoli
asthma
bronchial
cilia
common cold
COPD
cough
larynx
lower
pneumonia
pulmonary
respiration
rhinitis
sinuses
sinusitis
sneeze
surfactant
trachea
upper
ventilation

N	I	U	T	L	T	U	C	T	O	Y	T	H	I	S	E	D	R	A	T	S
T	S	R	R	E	S	P	I	R	A	T	I	O	N	B	S	A	A	D	N	A
E	E	S	U	C	L	R	U	A	N	P	F	Y	I	L	O	E	V	L	A	H
W	T	I	L	R	H	I	N	I	T	I	S	L	O	A	O	E	N	S	I	T
L	N	N	R	E	R	O	A	N	E	O	L	N	A	S	N	D	R	I	N	L
D	A	U	H	T	U	N	I	O	L	A	I	E	A	T	D	U	E	N	O	A
C	T	S	O	T	E	I	L	R	I	U	H	E	I	E	T	L	P	U	M	U
R	C	E	S	O	B	R	I	H	A	C	F	L	O	W	E	R	P	S	U	S
E	A	S	R	E	U	E	C	M	A	D	A	S	T	H	M	A	U	I	E	O
D	F	L	A	R	Y	N	X	R	P	T	D	H	E	G	A	A	L	T	N	D
I	R	R	Y	Z	O	P	T	O	I	N	E	U	H	U	L	B	Y	I	P	C
C	U	O	N	R	S	E	C	O	M	M	O	N	C	O	L	D	U	S	I	R
R	S	M	B	V	O	I	N	S	N	E	E	Z	E	C	R	I	E	S	T	A
O	M	A	P	U	L	M	O	N	A	R	Y	A	N	D	E	T	R	E	I	D
H	N	I	L	I	N	S	L	A	N	D	R	D	N	O	M	S	A	S	E	P

CHAPTER 54

Drugs Acting on the Upper Respiratory Tract

■ Crossword Puzzle

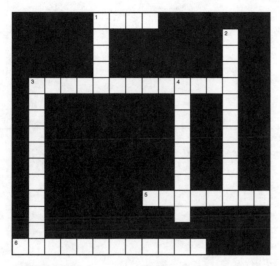

ACROSS

1 Common upper respiratory complaint caused by a virus
3 Drug that blocks the release of histamine and resultant vasodilation
5 Inflammation of the nares
6 Drug that stops membrane swelling and congestion

DOWN

1 Reflex to irritation in the upper respiratory tract
2 Drug that increases the cough reflex and removal of respiratory secretions
3 Drug that blocks the cough reflex
4 Drug that liquefies secretions in the respiratory tract

■ Web Exercise

R. W. recently moved to the area and has developed seasonal rhinitis. He had asthma as a child and is concerned that it might be returning. He asks for up-to-date information on the two disorders and how to survive the discomfort. Go to the Internet and find information that would be useful in preparing a teaching program for R. W.

■ Word Scramble

Unscramble the following letters to form the names of drugs commonly used to treat upper respiratory tract problems.

1. mactelseni _____

2. extramodernphhot _____

3. inpeerhed _____

4. hatzooterylriden _____

5. heednoripesuepd _____

6. dobnudesie _____

7. catflunusoe _____

8. mazetileso _____

■ Matching

Match the following drug names with the commonly used brand name.

1. _____ benzonatate
2. _____ azelastine
3. _____ chlorpheniramine
4. _____ cyproheptadine
5. _____ promethazine
6. _____ clemastine
7. _____ brompheniramine
8. _____ phenylephrine
9. _____ fluticasone
10. _____ budesonide

A. *Tavist*
B. *Flovent*
C. *Coricidin*
D. *Rhinocort*
E. *Tessalon*
F. *Dimetane*
G. *Astelin*
H. *Aller-Chlor*
I. *Phenergan*
J. *Periactin*

Drugs for Treating Obstructive Pulmonary Disorders

■ True or False

Indicate whether the following statements are true (T) or false (F).

_____ 1. Pulmonary obstructive diseases include asthma, emphysema, chronic obstructive pulmonary disease (COPD), respiratory distress syndrome, and seasonal rhinitis.

_____ 2. Drugs used to treat asthma and COPD include agents that block inflammation and dilate bronchi.

_____ 3. The xanthine derivatives have a direct effect on the smooth muscle of the respiratory tract.

_____ 4. The adverse effects of the xanthines are directly related to the theophylline levels and are fairly insignificant.

_____ 5. Sympathomimetics block the effects of the sympathetic nervous system and are used dilate the bronchi.

_____ 6. Anticholinergics can be used as bronchodilators because of their effect on the sympathetic nervous system receptor sites.

_____ 7. Steroids are used to decrease the inflammatory response in the airway.

_____ 8. Leukotriene receptor antagonists block or antagonize receptors for the production of leukotriene D_4 and E_4, thus blocking many of the signs and symptoms of asthma.

■ Web Exercise

You have a summer job as a nursing assistant and are required to have a physical and tuberculosis (TB) test. Having had many of these in the past, you are not concerned. However, the area on the arm that was injected becomes red and hard and is read as positive. You are very concerned and make an appointment at the health service for the next morning. Until then, you decide to find out all you can about this disease on the Internet to share with your family and roommates.

■ Word Search

Circle the names of the following drugs used to treat obstructive pulmonary disease that are hidden in the following grid. Words may appear diagonally, horizontally, or vertically.

aminophylline
caffeine
oxtriphylline
pentoxifylline
albuterol
isoproterenol
pirbuterol
ipratropium
flunisolide
zafirlukast
zileuton
cromolyn
nedocromil
beractant
colfosceril

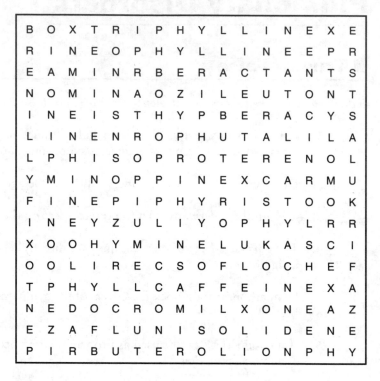

```
B O X T R I P H Y L L I N E X E
R I N E O P H Y L L I N E E P R
E A M I N R B E R A C T A N T S
N O M I N A O Z I L E U T O N T
I N E I S T H Y P B E R A C Y S
L I N E N R O P H U T A L I L A
L P H I S O P R O T E R E N O L
Y M I N O P P I N E X C A R M U
F I N E P I P H Y R I S T O O K
I N E Y Z U L I Y O P H Y L R R
X O O H Y M I N E L U K A S C I
O O L I R E C S O F L O C H E F
T P H Y L L C A F F E I N E X A
N E D O C R O M I L X O N E A Z
E Z A F L U N I S O L I D E N E
P I R B U T E R O L I O N P H Y
```

■ Word Scramble

Unscramble the following letters to form words related to lower respiratory tract diseases and therapies.

1. opehhytlelni _____

2. rotbullea _____

3. reeeppininh _____

4. trollmeesa _____

5. trappruimio _____

6. bedsudeion _____

7. firstluzkaa _____

8. tuzoline _____

9. tracbeant _____

10. cortapant _____

CHAPTER 56

Introduction to the Gastrointestinal System

■ Fill in the Blanks

Identify the parts of the gastrointestinal (GI) system in the following figure.

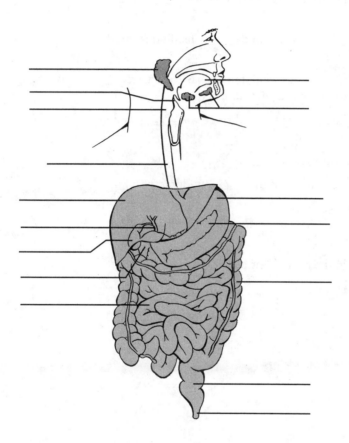

■ Matching

Match the following words with the appropriate definition.

1. _____ bile
2. _____ chyme
3. _____ gallstones
4. _____ gastrin
5. _____ histamine₂ receptors

A. Acid released in response to gastrin
B. Sites near the parietal cells of the stomach that cause the release of hydrochloric acid into the stomach.
C. Contents of the stomach
D. Pancreatin and pancrelipase
E. Network of nerve fibers running through the wall of the GI tract
F. Fluid stored in the gallbladder

6. _____ hydrochloric acid

7. _____ nerve plexus

8. _____ pancreatic enzymes

9. _____ peristalsis

10. _____ segmentation

G. Crystallization of cholesterol in the gallbladder

H. Secreted by the stomach to stimulate the release of hydrochloric acid

I. GI movement characterized by contraction of one segment of small intestine while the next segment is relaxed

J. GI movement characterized by a progressive wave of muscle contraction

■ Fill in the Blanks

1. The GI system is composed of one long tube and is responsible for _____ and _____ of nutrients.

2. Secretion of digestive enzymes, _____, bicarbonate, and _____ facilitates the digestion and absorption of nutrients.

3. The GI system is controlled by a(n) _____, which maintains a basic electrical rhythm and responds to local stimuli to increase or decrease activity.

4. The autonomic system can influence the activity of the GI tract; the _____ system slows it and the _____ system increases activity.

5. Initiation of activity in the GI tract depends on _____.

6. Overstimulation of any of the GI reflexes can result in _____ (underactivity) or _____ (overactivity).

7. Swallowing is a centrally mediated reflex that is important in delivering food to the GI tract for processing. It is controlled by the _____.

8. Vomiting is controlled by the _____ in the medulla or by the emetic zone in immature or injured brains.

■ Word Search

Circle the words related to the GI tract hidden in the following grid. Words may appear diagonally, horizontally, or vertically.

bile
chyme
emesis
esophagus
gallstones
gastrin
hydrochloric acid
local reflexes
mass movement
nerve plexus
pepsin
peristalsis
saliva
segmentation
stomach
sphincter
motility
vomiting
CTZ (chemoreceptor trigger zone)

D	A	R	V	C	O	R	T	U	P	O	M	H	I	W	N	S	S	B	R
A	S	P	H	I	N	C	T	E	R	N	L	A	T	S	I	D	R	A	E
L	I	T	H	N	I	O	T	A	T	N	E	M	G	E	S	I	T	V	E
E	W	S	U	X	E	L	P	E	V	R	E	N	R	A	C	C	E	O	S
D	E	E	P	P	E	T	B	N	R	D	S	P	B	Y	K	A	K	M	U
M	P	S	S	N	E	P	I	M	O	T	I	L	I	T	Y	C	T	I	M
A	E	O	C	C	E	R	T	U	E	T	E	P	E	P	S	I	N	T	E
N	R	P	O	S	T	U	I	N	A	U	L	M	E	H	E	R	E	I	E
D	I	H	R	S	A	G	A	S	A	L	I	V	A	S	R	O	M	N	R
M	S	A	A	G	A	L	L	S	T	O	N	E	S	R	S	L	E	G	H
I	T	G	E	F	A	W	S	P	N	A	H	O	H	E	T	H	V	T	S
N	A	U	R	Z	S	B	E	C	E	E	L	R	C	H	E	C	O	P	O
M	L	S	T	O	M	A	C	H	S	E	S	S	N	L	E	O	M	L	P
N	S	C	E	T	T	U	P	Y	C	E	I	P	I	U	W	R	S	L	O
A	I	A	L	C	N	R	S	M	P	S	E	B	R	S	I	D	S	R	E
E	S	T	O	H	I	M	E	E	M	E	S	I	S	C	X	Y	A	I	S
G	D	E	L	O	C	A	L	R	E	F	L	E	X	E	S	H	M	T	O
N	U	P	C	O	T	S	S	E	E	R	S	E	L	T	N	E	S	O	T

Drugs Affecting Gastrointestinal Secretions

■ Web Exercise

You are doing a rotation on medicine and working on a gastrointestinal (GI) unit. You are asked to prepare an inservice for the staff covering various GI diseases, treatments, and research and nursing implications involved in the care of patients with these disorders. Because this program will determine 20% of your course grade, you want to be current and thorough. Go to the Internet to prepare the teaching session.

■ Crossword Puzzle

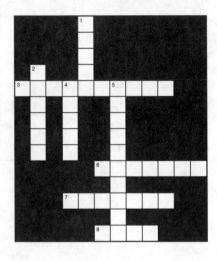

ACROSS

3 Digestive enzyme from the exocrine pancreas

6 Reflex increase in acid following a lowering of acid levels in the stomach

7 Digestive enzyme that results in the release of hydrochloric acid from cells in the stomach

8 Contributes to erosion of the stomach lining in peptic ulcer disease

DOWN

1 Erosion of the stomach or duodenal lining

2 Digestive and lubricating fluid in the mouth

4 Stomach contents

5 A drug that coats any injured area in the stomach

■ Matching

Match the following drugs with the appropriate class of drugs used to affect GI secretions. (Some classes may be used more than once.)

1. _____ misoprostol
2. _____ lansoprazole
3. _____ sucralfate
4. _____ cimetidine
5. _____ saliva
6. _____ aluminum
7. _____ sodium bicarbonate
8. _____ pancrelipase
9. _____ omeprazole
10. _____ famotidine

A. Histamine H_2 antagonists

B. Antacids

C. Proton pump inhibitors

D. Antipeptic agent

E. Prostaglandin

F. Digestive enzymes

■ Word Scramble

Unscramble the following letters to form the names of frequently used GI secretory agents.

1. faturscale _____
2. catparnine _____
3. mumnaliu _____
4. dimetincie _____
5. eesloomzeapr _____
6. valisa busttistue _____
7. daraaglemt _____
8. misoud aabbcinoret _____
9. midtoneifa _____
10. ooosstrpmil _____

CHAPTER 58

Laxatives and Antidiarrheal Agents

■ Patient Teaching Checklist

M. A. is a 55-year-old woman who has recently undergone a vaginal reconstruction. She is pain free and healing well but has become constipated and is afraid to move her bowels because of her fear of pain or ripping. An order is written for docusate. Prepare a drug teaching card for M. A. to take with her when she leaves.

■ Word Scramble

Unscramble the following letters to form the names of frequently used laxatives or antidiarrheal agents.

1. saccara _____

2. epromledia _____

3. discpaire _____

4. slyumipl _____

5. annse _____

6. romimcatpelode _____

7. umoip _____

8. ocatsude _____

■ True or False

Indicate whether the following statements are true (T) or false (F).

_____ 1. Laxatives are used to stop movement along the GI tract.

_____ 2. Laxatives are used to prevent or treat constipation.

_____ 3. Chemical stimulants directly irritate the local nerve plexus of the GI tract.

_____ 4. Bulk stimulants decrease the size of the food bolus and stimulate stretch receptors in the intestinal wall.

_____ 5. For many patients, eating a proper diet, exercising, and taking advantage of the actions of the intestinal reflexes has eliminated the need for laxatives.

_____ 6. Cathartic dependence can occur with the occasional use of laxatives, leading to a need for external stimuli for normal functioning of the GI tract.

_____ 7. GI stimulants act to increase sympathetic stimulation in the GI tract.

_____ 8. Antidiarrheal drugs are used to soothe irritation to the intestinal wall, block GI muscle activity to decrease movement, or affect central nervous system activity to cause GI spasm and stop movement.

■ Crossword Puzzle

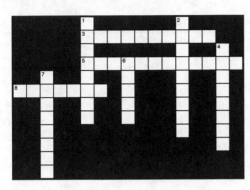

ACROSS

3 Antidiarrheal
5 Decreased GI activity
8 Chemical stimulant laxative

DOWN

1 Lubricant laxative
2 Chemical stimulant laxative; Dulcolax
4 Lubricant laxative; Colace
6 Chemical stimulant laxative; Senokot
7 Mild, bulk laxative

CHAPTER 59

Emetic and Antiemetic Agents

■ Listing

List four major contraindications for the induction of vomiting.

1. _____
2. _____
3. _____
4. _____

■ Crossword Puzzle

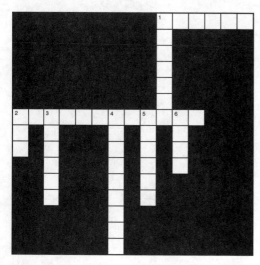

ACROSS

1 Protective response to vomiting reflex
2 Cancer treatment associated with nausea and vomiting

DOWN

1 Site of the CTZ
2 Chemoreceptor trigger zone
3 Inducing vomiting
4 Repetitive stimulation of the diaphragm

5 Vomiting is a centrally mediated _____
6 A common cause of nausea

■ Fill in the Blanks

1. Emetic drugs are used to induce _____ in cases of poisoning or drug overdose.

2. _____ is the standard antiemetic in use.

3. _____ are used to manage nausea and vomiting in situations in which they are not beneficial and could actually cause harm to the patient.

4. Antiemetics act by depressing the _____, either locally or through alteration of central nervous system actions.

5. Vomiting is a complex reflex mediated through the _____ located in the _____.

6. The chemoreceptor trigger zone (CTZ) can be stimulated by _____, _____, _____ or several other mechanisms.

7. Most antiemetics cause some _____, with resultant dizziness, drowsiness, and weakness.

8. _____ is another common adverse effect with antiemetics. Patients should be protected from exposure to the sun and ultraviolet light.

■ Word Search

Circle the names of commonly used antiemetic agents and related terms hidden in the following grid. Words may appear diagonally, horizontally, or vertically.

anticholinergics
antiemetic
buclizine
chlorpromazine
cyclizine
dolasetron
dronabinol
emetic
emetogenic
granisetron
hiccough
hydroxyzine
ipecac
metoclopramide
phenothiazine
photosensitivity
promethazine
vestibular

O	T	O	O	R	A	L	E	L	I	O	E	T	N	D	E	L	D	B	O	L	E
L	H	Y	D	R	O	X	Y	Z	I	N	E	Y	D	O	G	L	N	I	N	A	M
R	M	Y	R	I	L	L	K	Y	I	N	M	N	A	N	D	E	A	P	I	N	I
D	E	T	L	C	L	E	N	Z	R	R	E	O	E	A	R	I	K	H	S	T	H
O	T	I	O	T	H	R	I	A	M	I	T	M	C	L	O	L	R	E	A	I	S
T	O	V	R	A	I	L	D	D	D	C	I	A	N	D	N	E	A	N	N	C	E
L	C	I	A	D	C	V	O	I	K	H	C	A	O	K	A	E	M	O	N	H	C
Y	L	T	C	U	D	A	E	R	N	E	T	L	L	H	B	C	D	T	O	O	N
A	O	I	B	A	A	T	L	H	P	A	R	O	G	L	I	N	R	H	R	L	A
T	P	S	I	O	R	A	O	I	A	R	E	U	A	T	N	W	A	I	T	I	T
Y	R	N	H	S	M	N	R	U	S	R	O	N	E	A	O	U	L	A	E	N	S
T	A	E	N	I	Z	I	L	C	Y	C	L	M	M	D	L	R	U	Z	S	E	N
T	M	S	C	T	O	D	E	S	C	N	E	E	A	S	N	Z	B	I	I	R	A
O	I	O	N	C	N	T	S	I	O	I	L	C	Y	Z	A	E	I	N	N	G	P
R	D	T	A	A	O	A	H	T	T	D	U	A	D	I	I	R	T	E	A	I	A
A	E	O	I	R	L	K	K	N	R	F	F	R	U	R	L	N	S	O	R	C	I
C	A	H	B	D	O	L	A	S	E	T	R	O	N	U	E	J	E	C	G	S	C
T	N	P	E	O	E	M	E	T	O	G	E	N	I	C	N	O	V	R	L	R	T
T	C	Y	N	L	Y	B	R	L	E	N	I	Z	A	H	T	E	M	O	R	P	A
O	C	S	N	A	H	S	E	E	L	Y	Z	O	J	P	N	Y	A	E	M	I	P

Answer Key

Chapter 1: Introduction to Drugs

MATCHING
1. G   2. F   3. A   4. H   5. E   6. I   7. C   8. J   9. B   10. D

WEB EXERCISE
Start at http://www.fda.gov.

USE OF TERMS

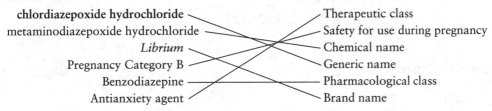

chlordiazepoxide hydrochloride — Therapeutic class
metaminodiazepoxide hydrochloride — Safety for use during pregnancy
Librium — Chemical name
Pregnancy Category B — Generic name
Benzodiazepine — Pharmacological class
Antianxiety agent — Brand name

DEFINITIONS
1. pharmacology: the study of the biological effects of chemicals
2. pharmacotherapeutics: clinical pharmacology, the branch of pharmacology involving drugs used to treat, prevent, or diagnose disease
3. genetic engineering: the process of altering deoxyribonucleic acid (DNA), which permits scientists to produce various drugs
4. preclinical trials: tests on laboratory animals of chemicals that may have therapeutic value
5. generic name: the original designation that the drug is given when the drug company applies for the approval process
6. orphan drugs: drugs that have been discovered but that are not financially viable and therefore have not been "adopted" by any drug company
7. over-the-counter (OTC) drugs: products that are available without prescriptions for self-treatment of a variety of complaints
8. FDA pregnancy category: a rating that will indicate the potential or actual teratogenic effects of a drug

FILL IN THE BLANKS

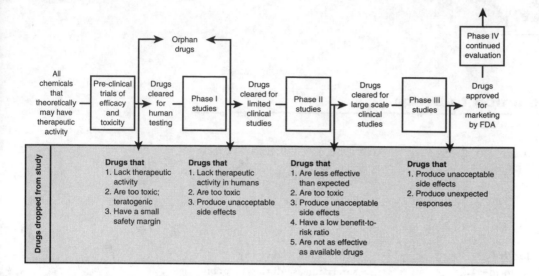

Chapter 2: Drugs and the Body

WORD SEARCH

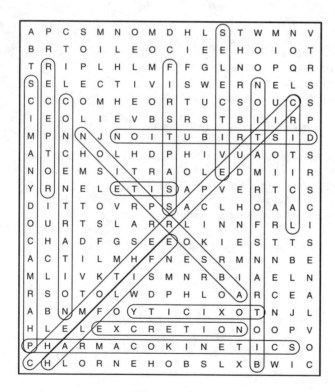

FILL IN THE BLANKS

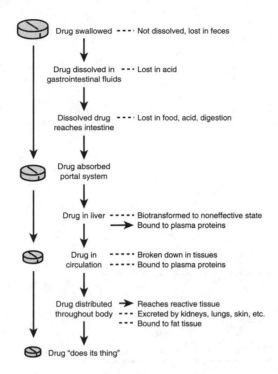

Drug swallowed ---- Not dissolved, lost in feces

Drug dissolved in --- Lost in acid
gastrointestinal fluids

Dissolved drug --- Lost in food, acid, digestion
reaches intestine

Drug absorbed
portal system

Drug in liver ----- Biotransformed to noneffective state
→ Bound to plasma proteins

Drug in ----- Broken down in tissues
circulation ----- Bound to plasma proteins

Drug distributed → Reaches reactive tissue
throughout body --- Excreted by kidneys, lungs, skin, etc.
--- Bound to fat tissue

Drug "does its thing"

MULTIPLE CHOICE

1. c   2. c   3. b   4. d   5. b   6. c   7. b   8. d

WORD SCRAMBLE

1. biotransformation
2. distribution
3. placebo
4. excretion
5. pharmacokinetics
6. receptor sites
7. half life
8. chemotherapeutic

Chapter 3: Toxic Effects of Drugs

DEFINITIONS

1. anaphylactic reaction: an allergy involving an antibody that reacts with specific sites in the body to cause the release of chemicals, including histamine, that produce immediate reactions—mucous membrane swelling and constricting bronchi—that can lead to respiratory distress and even respiratory arrest
2. cytotoxic reaction: an allergy involving antibodies that circulate in the blood and attack antigens (the drug) on cell sites, causing death of that cell. This reaction is not immediate but may be seen over a few days.
3. serum sickness reaction: an allergy involving antibodies that circulate in the blood and cause damage to various tissues by depositing in blood vessels. This reaction may occur up to a week or more after exposure to the drug.
4. superinfection: infections caused by the destruction of normal flora bacteria by certain drugs, allowing other bacteria to enter the body and cause infection
5. blood dyscrasia: bone marrow depression caused by drug effects that occur when drugs that can cause cell death (antineoplastics, antibiotics) are used

6. hypersensitivity reaction: when a patient exhibits excessive response to either the primary or the secondary effects of a drug
7. stomatitis: inflammation of the mucous membranes with swollen gums, swollen and red tongue, difficulty breathing, and pain in the mouth and throat

MATCHING

1. E   2. C   3. A   4. F   5. B   6. D

FILL IN THE BLANKS

1. gentamicin
2. hypoglycemia
3. chloroquine
4. auditory damage
5. blood dyscrasia
6. dizziness and drowsiness

Chapter 4: Nursing Management

LISTING

1. Drug
2. Storage
3. Route
4. Dosage
5. Preparation
6. Timing
7. Recording

FILL IN THE BLANKS

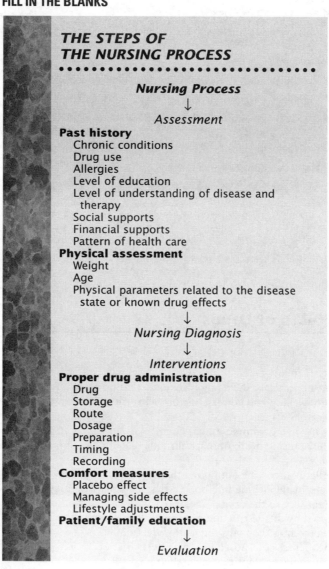

THE STEPS OF THE NURSING PROCESS

Nursing Process
↓
Assessment

Past history
  Chronic conditions
  Drug use
  Allergies
  Level of education
  Level of understanding of disease and therapy
  Social supports
  Financial supports
  Pattern of health care
Physical assessment
  Weight
  Age
  Physical parameters related to the disease state or known drug effects
↓
Nursing Diagnosis
↓
Interventions
Proper drug administration
  Drug
  Storage
  Route
  Dosage
  Preparation
  Timing
  Recording
Comfort measures
  Placebo effect
  Managing side effects
  Lifestyle adjustments
Patient/family education
↓
Evaluation

LISTING

1. Name, dose, and action of drug
2. Timing of administration
3. Special storage and preparation
4. Specific OTC drugs to avoid
5. Special comfort or safety measures
6. Safety measures
7. Specific points about drug toxicity
8. Specific warnings about drug discontinuation

Chapter 5: Dosage Calculations

MATCHING

1. E   2. A   3. F   4. C   5. D   6. B

DOSAGE CALCULATIONS

1. a. 0.1 g
   b. 1.5 kg
   c. 100 mL
   d. 0.5 L
2. a. 9 g
   b. 15 mg
   c. 3 mL
   d. 2 L
3. a. 1 tsp
   b. 2 tbs
4. a. 77 kg
   b. 7 lb
5. 11.25 mL
6. 3.3 mL
7. a. 2 capsules
   b. 500 mg
8. 15 mg
9. 6 mL
10. a. two; one
    b. 1500 mg
11. 0.65 mL
12. 0.58 (0.6) mL
13. 1.6 mL
14. 1.9 mL
15. 1.5 mL
16. 3 mL
17. 2.4 mL
18. 0.5 mL
19. 125 mL/hr; 13 drops/min
20. 125 mL/hr; 21 drops/min

MULTIPLE CHOICE

1. d   2. c   3. d   4. b   5. b   6. b   7. d   8. b

Chapter 6: Drug Therapy in the 21st Century

MATCHING

1. C   2. D   3. A   4. E   5. A   6. E   7. A   8. C   9. B   10. B

WORD SEARCH

```
A S D A N D E L I O N O B E K J I L M O R
B K O L E A N D G I N K O B E L I O N F S
O A L O E K A V I L S M R I E P H E D R A
S V A L E R I A N P E U C A L Y P T U S W
A A I I P O C H S H C H C H I C O R Y A P
W S L C H S H R E E S I L E M L R I L W A
A P I O O E N M N B I O N D O A N D A P L
S I L R O M A R G I N G E R M E S L E E M
L M S I V A L F A L F A V A A L O I R P E
I S L C K R P T D B L A C K C O H O S H T
N O M E O Y O K I E C H I N A C E A H R T
G E R C F E N U G R E E K I Y U Y U N L O
O D O H U R T A R R A G O N H S P L R T N
L D S I N G R E E Y R N M K N L T I L O S
```

DEFINITIONS

1. self-care: tendency for patients to self-diagnose and determine their own treatment needs
2. Internet: the worldwide digital information system accessed through computer systems
3. OTC drugs: drugs that are available without a prescription for self-treatment of a variety of complaints
4. alternative therapies: including herbs and other "natural" products as found in ancient records, these products are not controlled or tested by the Food and Drug Administration (FDA) and because of this, the advertising surrounding these products is not as restricted or accurate as it would be with classic drugs
5. off-label uses: when a drug is approved by the FDA, the therapeutic indications for which the drug is approved are stated; once a drug is available, that drug often is used for indications that are not part of the approved indications, these are called off-label uses
6. cost comparisons: a comparison of the relative cost of the same drug provided by different manufacturers to determine the costs to the consumer

Chapter 7: Introduction to Cell Physiology

WEB EXERCISE

Follow online instructions.

FILL IN THE BLANKS

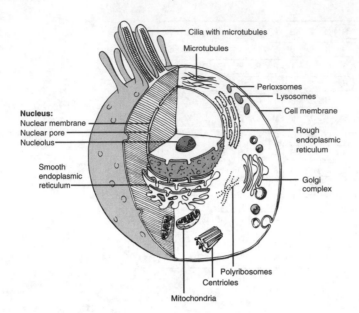

WORD SCRAMBLE

1. diffusion
2. endocytosis
3. pinocytosis
4. phagocytosis
5. osmosis
6. mitosis
7. passive transport
8. active transport

MATCHING

1. E   2. D   3. B   4. C   5. A

CROSSWORD PUZZLE

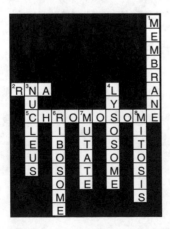

Chapter 8: Anti-infective Agents

DEFINITIONS

1. culture: sample of the bacteria (eg, from sputum, cell scrapings, urine) to grow in a laboratory to determine the species of bacteria that is causing an infection

2. prophylaxis: treatment to prevent an infection before it occurs, as in the use of antibiotics to prevent disease such as bacterial endocarditis or antiprotozoals to prevent malaria

3. resistance: ability of bacteria over time to adapt to an antibiotic and produce cells that are no longer affected by the drug

4. selective toxicity: property of antibiotics that allows them to affect certain proteins or enzyme systems that are used by bacteria but not by human cells, sparing the human cells from the destructive effects of the antibiotic

5. sensitivity testing: evaluation of bacteria obtained in a culture to determine to what antibiotics the organisms are sensitive and which agent would be appropriate for treatment of a particular infection

6. spectrum: range of bacteria against which an antibiotic is effective (eg, broad-spectrum antibiotics are effective against a wide range of bacteria)

CROSSWORD PUZZLE

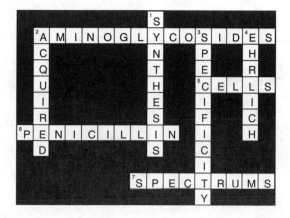

MATCHING

1. C   2. A   3. B   4. E   5. F   6. D

MULTIPLE CHOICE

1. c   2. d   3. a   4. b   5. c

Chapter 9: Antibiotics

TRUE OR FALSE

1. T
2. F
3. F
4. T
5. F
6. T
7. F
8. T

WEB EXERCISE

Use www.cdc.gov to obtain the information. Development of the information will be individual.

WORD SCRAMBLE

1. cephapirin
2. cefaclor
3. cefadroxil
4. loracarbef
5. ceftizoxime
6. cefotetan
7. cefoxitin
8. cefazolin

MATCHING

1. G   2. F   3. I   4. A   5. B   6. J   7. C   8. D   9. E
10. C   11. A   12. H

Chapter 10: Antiviral Agents

IDENTIFY SITE OF ACTION

1. Reverse transcriptase inhibitors bind directly to HIV to reverse transcriptase, which blocks both ribonucleic acid- (RNA) and DNA-dependent DNA polymerase activities. This prevents the transfer of information that would allow the virus to replicate and survive.
2. Protease inhibitors block protease, which is essential for the maturation of infectious virus, within the HIV virus; an immature and noninfective virus is produced.
3. Nucleosides inhibit HIV replication by inhibiting cell protein synthesis, leading to viral death.
4. Antiretrovirus drugs act to prevent replication in various retroviruses, including HIV; action is related to their conversion to triphosphates in the body.

MATCHING

1. F   2. D   3. E   4. C   5. A   6. B

WORD SCRAMBLE

1. famciclovir
2. oseltamivir
3. ganciclovir
4. rimantadine
5. acyclovir
6. valacyclovir
7. amantadine
8. ribavirin
9. foscarnet
10. zanamivir
11. valganciclovir
12. cidofovir

PATIENT TEACHING CHECKLIST

ZIDOVUDINE

An antiviral works in combination with other antivirals to stop the replication of the AIDS virus and to maintain the functioning of your immune system.

This drug is not a cure for AIDS or an AIDS-related complex (ARC); opportunistic infections may occur and regular medical follow-up should be sought to deal with the disease.

This drug does not reduce the risk of transmission of HIV to others by sexual contact or by blood contamination; use appropriate precautions.

Common effects of this drug include:

- Dizziness, weakness, loss of feeling—Change positions slowly; if you feel drowsy, avoid driving or performing dangerous activities.
- Headache, fever, muscle aches—Analgesics may be ordered to alleviate this discomfort. Consult with your health care provider.
- Nausea, loss of appetite, change in taste—Small, frequent meals may help. It is important to try to maintain your nutrition. Consult your health care provider if this becomes a severe problem.

Report any of the following to your health care provider: excessive fatigue, lethargy, severe headache, difficulty breathing, skin rash.

Avoid over-the-counter (OTC) medications. If you feel that you need one of these, check with your health care provider first.

Regular medical evaluations, including blood tests, will be needed to monitor the effects of these drugs on your body and to adjust dosages as needed.

Tell any doctor, nurse, or other health care provider that you are taking these drugs.

Keep this drug, and all medications, out of the reach of children. Do not share these drugs with other people.

FILL IN THE BLANKS

1. zanamivir
2. ribavirin
3. amantadine
4. foscarnet
5. valacyclovir
6. acyclovir
7. zidovudine
8. penciclovir

Chapter 11: Antifungal Agents

WEB EXERCISE

Looking up both Internet sources will provide patient teaching materials that can be organized into a usable format.

WORD SEARCH

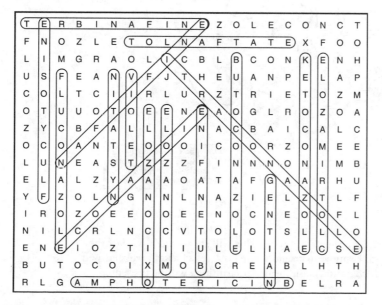

FILL IN THE BLANKS

1. hard, ergosterol
2. mycosis
3. hepatic, renal
4. Candida
5. tinea
6. systemically
7. wounds
8. burning, irritation, pain

MATCHING

1. B   2. C   3. A   4. D   5. H   6. F   7. G   8. E

Chapter 12: Antiprotozoal Agents

MATCHING

1. D   2. E   3. B   4. F   5. A   6. G   7. C

FILL IN THE BLANKS

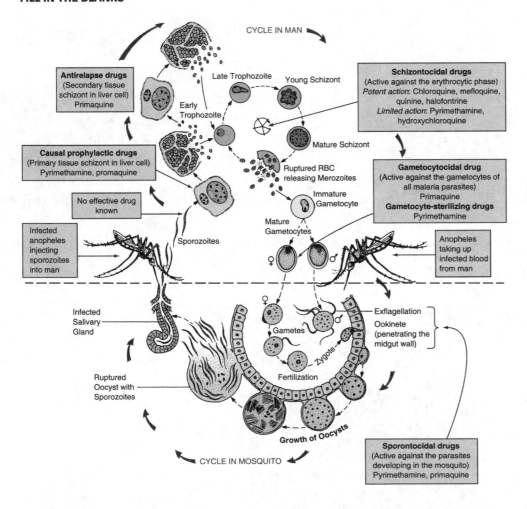

WEB EXERCISE

Go to www.cdc.gov/travel. Select the graphic travel map. This will show you a map of the world with certain areas highlighted. Using your friend's itinerary, select each area that will be visited. Health risks, suggested vaccinations, and health precautions will be presented (and can be printed). Back on the home page, you can select summary sheets for travel hazards, precautions, and even areas of unrest and political precautions.

MATCHING

1. A   2. B   3. A   4. C   5. A   6. A   7. D   8. A

Chapter 13: Anthelmintic Agents

DEFINITIONS

1. cestode: tapeworm with a head and segmented body parts that is capable of growing to several yards in the human intestine
2. nematode: roundworm such as the commonly encountered pinworm, whipworm, threadworm, *Ascaris,* or hookworm
3. pinworm: nematode that causes a common helmintic infection in humans; lives in the intestine and causes anal and possible vaginal irritation and itching
4. round worm: worm such as *Ascaris* that causes a common helmintic infection in humans; can cause intestinal obstruction because the adult worms clog the intestinal lumen or severe pneumonia when the larvae migrate to the lungs and form a pulmonary infiltrate
5. schistosomiasis: infection with blood fluke that is carried by a snail, poses a common problem in tropical countries, where the snail is the intermediary in the life cycle of the worm; larvae burrow into the skin in fresh water and migrate throughout the human body, causing a rash and then symptoms of diarrhea and liver and brain inflammation
6. trichinosis: disease that results from ingestion of encysted roundworm larvae in undercooked pork; larvae migrate throughout the body to invade muscle and nervous tissue; can cause pneumonia, heart failure, and encephalitis
7. thread worm: pervasive nematode that can send larvae into the lungs, liver, and central nervous system (CNS); can cause severe pneumonia or liver abscess
8. whip worm: worm that attaches itself to the intestinal mucosa and sucks blood; may cause severe anemia and disintegration of the intestinal mucosa

PATIENT TEACHING CHECKLIST

MEBENDAZOLE

An anthelmintic acts to destroy certain helminths or worms that have invaded your body. You must take the full course of the drug that has been prescribed for you to ensure that you have cleared all of the worms, in all phases of their life cycle, from your body. Your drug has been prescribed to treat pinworms.

Your drug can be taken with meals or with a light snack to help decrease any stomach upset that you may experience.

Common effects of this drug include:

- Nausea, vomiting, loss of appetite—Take the drug with meals and eat small, frequent meals.
- Dizziness, drowsiness—If this happens, avoid driving a car or operating dangerous machinery; change positions slowly to avoid falling or injury.

Report any of the following to your health care provider: fever, chills, rash, headache, weakness, or tremors.

It is very important to take the complete prescription that has been ordered for you. Never use this drug to self-treat any other infection or give it to any other person.

Tell any doctor, nurse, or other health care provider that you are taking this drug.

Keep this drug, and all medications, out of the reach of children.

Follow the following guidelines to help to prevent reinfection with the worms or spread to other family members:

- Wash hands vigorously with soap after using toilet facilities.
- Shower in the morning to wash away any ova deposited in the anal area during the night.
- Change and launder undergarments, bed linens, and pajamas every day.
- Disinfect toilets and toilet seats daily and bathroom and bedroom floors periodically.

FILL IN THE BLANKS

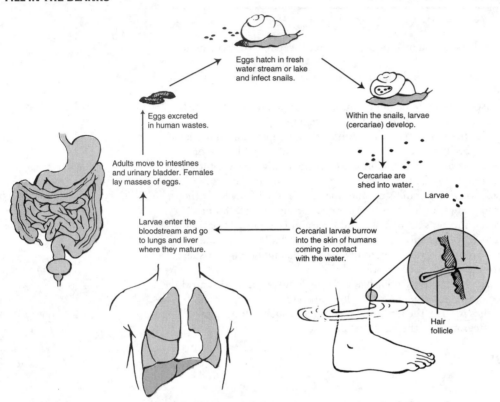

WORD SEARCH

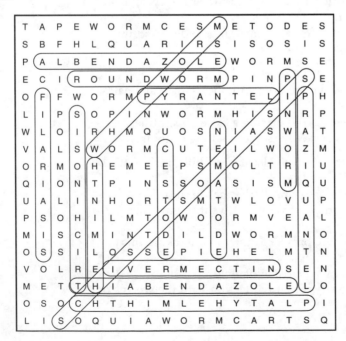

Chapter 14: Antineoplastic Agents

NURSING CARE GUIDE

Busulfan

Assessment	Nursing Diagnoses	Implementation	Evaluation
HISTORY Allergies to busulfan, renal or liver dysfunction, pregnancy and lactation, bone marrow depression, GI ulceration	Acute pain related to GI, CNS, skin effects Impaired nutrition related to GI effects Impaired self-concept related to diagnosis, therapy, side effects Deficient knowledge regarding drug therapy	Ensure safe preparation and administration of the drug. Provide comfort and safety measures: -mouth and skin care -rest periods -safety precautions -antiemetics as needed -maintenance of nutrition -head covering. Provide small, frequent meals and monitor nutritional status. Provide support and reassurance to deal with drug effects, discomfort, and diagnosis. Provide patient teaching regarding drug name, dosage, adverse effects, precautions, warnings to report, and comfort measures to observe.	Evaluate drug effects: resolution of cancer being treated. Monitor for adverse effects: -GI toxicity -bone marrow depression -CNS changes -renal, hepatic damage -alopecia -extravasation of drug. Evaluate effectiveness of patient teaching program. Evaluate effectiveness of comfort and safety measures.
PHYSICAL EXAMINATION Local: injection site evaluation CNS: orientation, affect, reflexes Skin: color, lesions, texture GI: abdominal, liver evaluation Hematological: renal and hepatic function tests, CBC with differential			

MATCHING

1. D   2. G   3. C   4. E   5. F   6. A   7. H   8. B

WORD SCRAMBLE

1. vinblastine
2. carmustine
3. carboplatin
4. cisplatin
5. tamoxifen
6. bleomycin
7. dacarbazine
8. etoposide

FILL IN THE BLANKS

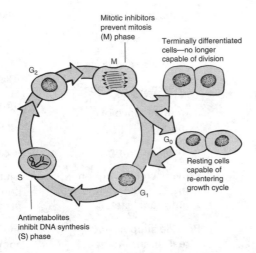

CROSSWORD PUZZLE

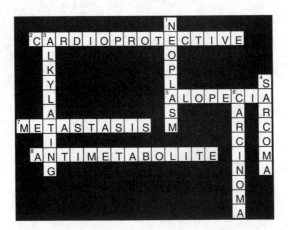

Chapter 15: Introduction to the Immune Response and Inflammation

MULTIPLE CHOICE

1. d   2. c   3. a   4. b   5. a   6. c

FILL IN THE BLANKS

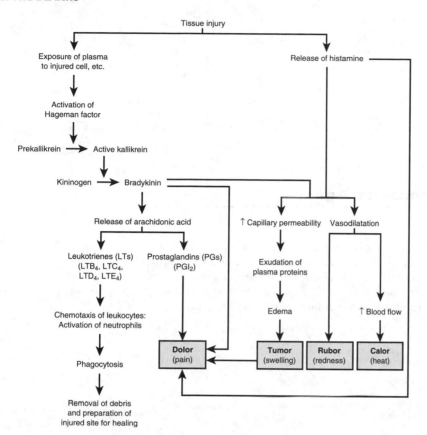

WORD SEARCH

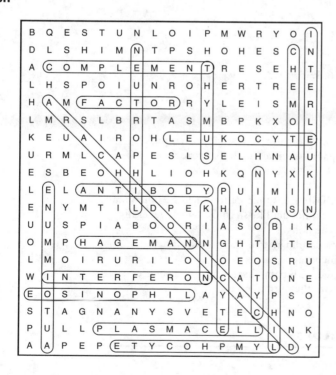

TRUE OR FALSE

1. T
2. F
3. T
4. F
5. F
6. F
7. F
8. T
9. F
10. T

Chapter 16: Anti-inflammatory Agents

WEB EXERCISE

Go to http://www.arthritis.org. At the top of the home page is a "search" slot where you can enter any key word—research, drugs, etc. Or you can select the menu under "Offerings" and select "What's new," "Order brochures," or "Getting a Grip on Rheumatoid Arthritis." You can also go to the lower part of the home page and find local groups that might be appropriate for your patient as support groups, exercise groups, or information sources.

WORD SCRAMBLE

1. naproxen
2. sulindac
3. ketorolac
4. diclofenac
5. ibuprofen
6. olsalazine
7. acetaminophen
8. salsalate
9. aspirin
10. ketoprofen

MATCHING

1. D   2. G   3. E   4. C   5. B   6. F   7. A

DEFINITIONS

1. analgesic: an agent used to decrease pain
2. anti-inflammatory: an agent that blocks the inflammatory reaction, preventing or decreasing the swelling, redness, heat, and pain associated with that reaction
3. antipyretic: an agent used to decrease fever
4. chrysotherapy: treatment with gold salts
5. nonsteroidal anti-inflammatory drugs (NSAIDs): drugs that act to block the inflammatory reaction at the site of the reaction; they do not act like steroids, which generally block the inflammatory system throughout the body
6. salicylates: drugs that act to block the prostaglandin system and prevent inflammation and therefore pain, fever, and discomfort; includes aspirin
7. arthritis: inflammation of the joints associated with pain, disability, and disfigurement
8. fever: elevation of the body temperature above the normal range

Chapter 17: Immune Modulators

DEFINITIONS

1. autoimmune: having antibodies to self-cells or self-proteins; leads to chronic inflammatory disease and cell destruction

2. interferon: protein released by cells in response to viral invasion; prevents viral replication in other cells
3. interleukin: "between white cells"; substance released by active white cells to communicate with other white cells and to support the inflammatory and immune reactions
4. monoclonal antibodies: specific antibodies produced by a single clone of B cells to react with a specific antigen
5. immune suppressant: drug used to block or suppress the actions of the T cells and antibody production; used to prevent transplant rejection and treat autoimmune diseases

MATCHING

1. E   2. B   3. F   4. G   5. A   6. C   7. D

FILL IN THE BLANKS

1. Monoclonal antibodies
2. basiliximab, daclizumab, muromonab-CD3
3. Crohn's
4. respiratory syncytial virus
5. trastuzumab
6. Rituximab
7. omalizumb
8. alemtuzumab

WORD SEARCH

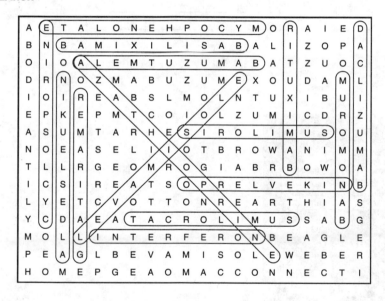

Chapter 18: Vaccines and Sera

WEB EXERCISE

Go to http://www.aap.org/family/parents/vaccine.htm. This page, maintained by the American Academy of Pediatrics, can be printed out and offers answers to the most frequently asked parent questions about vaccinations. A permanent record of vaccinations can be printed out from the bottom of the page if other forms are not available.

TRUE OR FALSE

1. F
2. T
3. T
4. T
5. T
6. T
7. F
8. F

FILL IN THE BLANKS
Recommended Immunication Schedule, Pediatric

Vaccine	Birth	2 mo	4 mo	6 mo	12 mo	15 mo	18 mo	24 mo	4–6 y	11–12 y	14–16 y
Hepatitis B		X	X			X				0	
Hepatitis B*	X	X		X							
DPT		X	X	X			X		X		
Tetanus Booster									X		X
H. influenzae b		X	X	X	X						
Poliovirus (IPV)		X	X		X				X		
Measles, mumps, rubella					X				X	0	
Varicella						X				0	
Hepatitis A†									X		

0—suggested timing of immunization if recommended immunizations have been missed, or given early.
* Infants born to HBsAg-positive mothers.
† Recommended in selected areas only, check with your local Health Department.
Suggested by the American Academy of Pediatrics, January, 2000

CROSSWORD PUZZLE

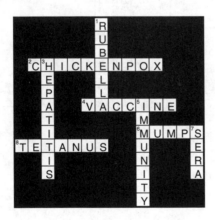

Chapter 19: Introduction to Nerves and the Nervous System

LABELING

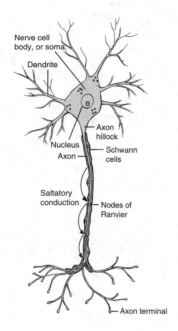

Nerve cell body, or soma

Dendrite

Axon hillock

Nucleus

Axon

Schwann cells

Saltatory conduction

Nodes of Ranvier

Axon terminal

MATCHING

1. G   2. C   3. B   4. J   5. I   6. H   7. A   8. F   9. E   10. D

DIAGRAM

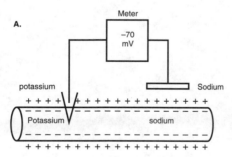

A.

Meter

−70 mV

potassium

Sodium

+ + + + + + + + + + + + + + + + + +

Potassium

sodium

– – – – – – – – – – – – – – – – – – –

+ + + + + + + + + + + + + + + + + + +

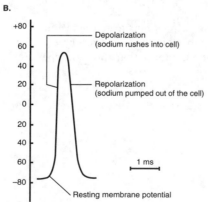

B.

+80
60
40
20
0
20
40
60
−80

Depolarization (sodium rushes into cell)

Repolarization (sodium pumped out of the cell)

1 ms

Resting membrane potential

WORD SEARCH

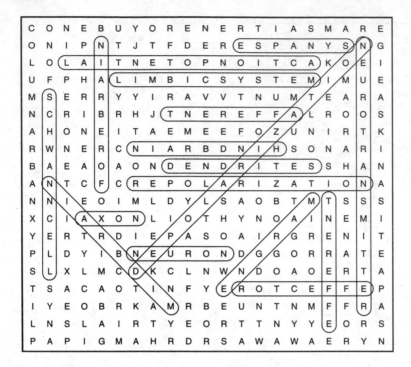

Chapter 20: Anxiolytic and Hypnotic Agents

FILL IN THE BLANKS

1. Anxiety
2. motivator
3. Sedatives
4. hypnotics
5. tension, fear
6. sedation
7. depress
8. Benzodiazepines

MATCHING

1. C   2. E   3. A   4. B   5. G   6. H   7. D   8. F   9. J   10. I

WEB EXERCISE

Go to http://www.adaa.org. Select "Public," then select Self-Help Groups from the menu. Select your state and locate support groups in your area. Go back to the public resource page and select "Anxiety Disorders Information" and print out information about the specific anxiety diagnosis related to this patient.

WORD SCRAMBLE

1. benzodiazepine
2. hypnotic
3. sedative
4. barbiturate
5. buspirone
6. zaleplon
7. zolpidem
8. diazepam
9. phenobarbital
10. anxiolytic

Chapter 21: Antidepressant Agents

MULTIPLE CHOICE

1. a   2. b   3. b   4. c   5. c

WORD SEARCH

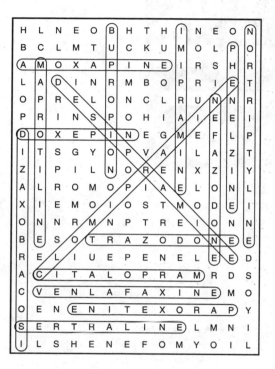

WORD SCRAMBLE

1. bupropion
2. fluoxetine
3. clomipramine
4. venlafaxine
5. phenelzine
6. paroxetine
7. imipramine
8. nefazodone

CROSSWORD PUZZLE

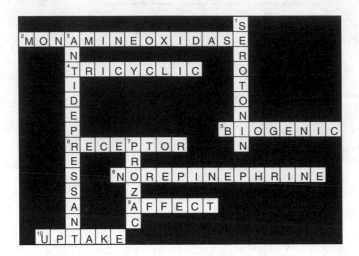

FILL IN THE BLANKS

1. norepinephrine, dopamine, serotonin
2. breakdown, synaptic cleft
3. reuptake
4. norepinephrine, serotonin
5. tyramine
6. PMDD (premenstrual dysphoric disorder)
7. Bupropion
8. anticholinergic

Chapter 22: Psychotherapeutic Agents

MATCHING

1. F   2. C   3. B   4. G   5. D   6. A   7. E

PATIENT TEACHING CHECKLIST

CHLORPROMAZINE

An antipsychotic or a neuroleptic drug that affects the activities of certain chemicals in your brain and is used to treat certain mental disorders.

The drug should be taken exactly as prescribed. Because this drug also affects many body systems, it is important that you have regular medical evaluation.

Common effects of these drugs include:

- Dizziness, drowsiness, fainting—Avoid driving or performing hazardous tasks or delicate tasks that require concentration if these occur. Change position slowly. The dizziness usually passes after 1 to 2 weeks of drug use.
- Pink or reddish urine—Do not be alarmed by this change; it does not mean that your urine contains blood. The drug causes some people's urine to change to this color.
- Sensitivity to light—Bright light might hurt your eyes, and sunlight might burn your skin more easily. Wear sunglasses and protective clothing when you must be out in the sun.
- Constipation—Consult with your health care provider if this becomes a problem.

Report any of the following to your health care provider: sore throat, fever, rash; tremors, weakness; vision changes.

Tell any doctor, nurse, or other health care provider that you are taking this drug.

Keep this drug, and all medications, out of the reach of children.

Avoid the use of alcohol or other depressants when you are taking this drug. You also may want to limit your use of caffeine if you have increased tension or insomnia.

Avoid the use of over-the-counter (OTC) drugs when you are taking this drug. Many of them contain ingredients that could interfere with the effectiveness of the drug. If you believe that you need one of these preparations, consult with your health care provider about the most appropriate choice.

Take this drug exactly as prescribed. If you run out of medicine or find that you cannot take your drug for any reason, consult your health care provider. After the drug has been used for a period of time, there is a risk of adverse effects if the drug is suddenly stopped. This drug must be tapered over time.

Specifics related to your situation: You must be very careful about driving, especially during the first few weeks of treatment. Use sunscreen and protective clothing whenever you are outside and use sunglasses.

WEB EXERCISE

Go to http://www.mhsource.com. Select Disorders from the pull-down menu under Resources. Read the Ask the Expert information under Seasonal Affective Disorder to learn about treatment options—herbal and alternative therapies and light therapy, including insurance backing of the purchase of lights.

WORD SCRAMBLE

1. molindone
2. pimozide
3. ziprasidone
4. thiothixene
5. risperidone
6. mesoridazine
7. loxapine
8. haloperidol
9. triflupromazine
10. clozapine

Chapter 23: Antiepileptic Agents

FILL IN THE BLANKS

1. Epilepsy
2. seizure
3. convulsion
4. antiepileptics
5. grand mal seizure
6. absence seizure
7. myoclonic seizures
8. febrile seizures
9. status epilepticus
10. focal

NURSING CARE GUIDE

Hydantoin

Assessment	Nursing Diagnoses	Implementation	Evaluation
HISTORY Allergies to any of these drugs; hypotension; arrhythmias, bone marrow depression, coma, psychoses, pregnancy and lactation, hepatic or renal dysfunction	Acute pain related to GI, CNS, GU effects High risk for injury related to CNS effects Disturbed thought processes related to CNS effects Deficient knowledge regarding drug therapy Alteration in skin integrity related to dermatological effects	Discontinue drug at first sign of liver dysfunction, skin rash Provide comfort and safety measures: -positioning -give with meals -safety measures -barrier contraceptives -skin care Provide support and reassurance to deal with diagnosis and drug effects Provide patient teaching regarding drug, dosage, drug effects, things to report, need to wear medical alert information	Evaluate drug effects: decrease in incidence and frequency of seizures. Monitor for adverse effects: -CNS effects—multiple -bone marrow depression -rash, skin changes -GI effects—nausea, anorexia -arrhythmias Monitor for drug–drug interactions: Increased depression with CNS depressant, alcohol; varies with individual drug. Evaluate effectiveness of patient teaching program. Evaluate effectiveness of comfort and safety measures.
PHYSICAL EXAMINATION CV: BP, P, peripheral perfusion CNS: orientation, affect, reflexes, strength, EEG Skin: color, lesions, texture, temperature GI: abdominal exam, bowel sounds Resp: R, adventitious sounds Other: renal and liver function tests			

CROSSWORD PUZZLE

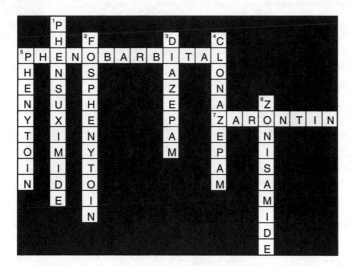

WORD SEARCH

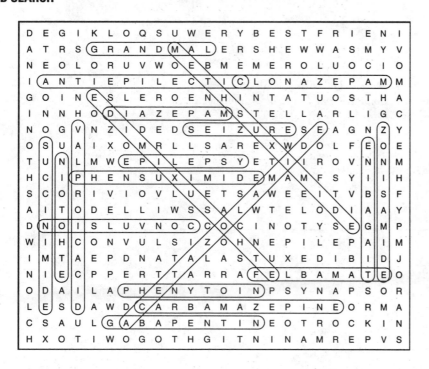

Chapter 24: Antiparkinsonism Agents

FILL IN THE BLANKS

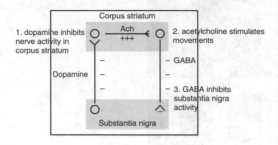

WORD SCRAMBLE

1. levodopa
2. procyclidine
3. pergolide
4. biperiden
5. amantadine
6. ropinirole
7. benztropine
8. bromocriptine

WEB EXERCISE

Go to http://www.ninds.nih.gov. From the Disorders Quick Links pull-down menu, select Parkinson's. Choose topics from the Information Page that would be of interest to this family—research, surgery, support groups, etc.

MULTIPLE CHOICE

1. b   2. d   3. c   4. a   5. c   6. b   7. d   8. a

Chapter 25: Muscle Relaxants

MATCHING

1. C   2. E   3. H   4. F   5. A   6. B   7. G   8. D

FILL IN THE BLANKS

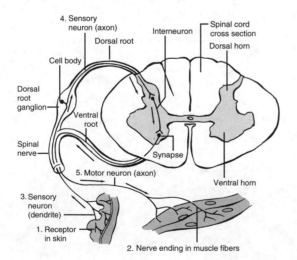

TRUE OR FALSE

1. F
2. T
3. F
4. F
5. T
6. F
7. T
8. F
9. T
10. T

CROSSWORD PUZZLE

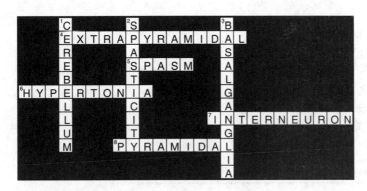

Chapter 26: Narcotics and Antimigraine Agents

WORD SEARCH

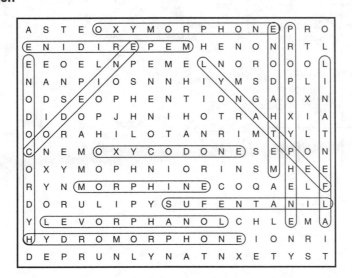

MATCHING

1. G   2. F   3. D   4. H   5. J   6. C   7. B   8. I   9. E   10. A

MULTIPLE CHOICE

1. a   2. b   3. b   4. c   5. a

DEFINITIONS

1. A fibers: large-diameter nerve fibers that carry peripheral impulses associated with touch and temperature to the spinal cord
2. A-delta and C fibers: small-diameter nerve fibers that carry peripheral impulses associated with pain to the spinal cord
3. gate-control theory: theory that the transmission of nerve impulses can be modulated at several points along its path by the closing and opening of "gates"
4. migraine headache: headache characterized by severe, unilateral, pulsating head pain and associated with systemic effects, including gastrointestinal (GI) upset, light and sound sensitization
5. narcotics: drugs originally derived from opium that react with specific opioid receptors in the body
6. narcotic agonists: drugs that act at opioid receptors to stimulate the effects of the receptors
7. narcotic agonists–antagonists: drugs that act at some opioid receptors to stimulate activity and at other opioid receptors to block activity
8. narcotic antagonists: drugs that block opioid receptors, used to counteract the effects of narcotics and to treat narcotic overdoses
9. opioid receptors: receptor sites on nerves that react with enkephalins and endorphins and that are receptive to narcotic drugs
10. triptan: selective serotonin receptor blocker that causes a vascular constriction of cranial vessels, used to treat acute migraine attacks

Chapter 27: General and Local Anesthetic Agents

FILL IN THE BLANKS

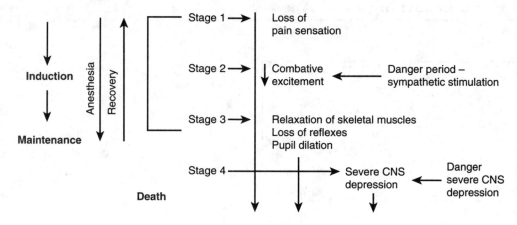

NURSING CARE GUIDE

Local Anesthetic

Assessment	Nursing Diagnoses	Implementation	Evaluation
HISTORY Allergies to any of these drugs, parabens; cardiac disorders; vascular problems; hepatic dysfuntion	Impaired perception related to anesthetic High risk for injury related to loss of sensation, mobility Alteration in skin integrity related to immobility Deficient knowledge regarding drug therapy	Ensure administration of drug under strict supervision Provide comfort and safety measures: -positioning -skin care -side rails -pain medication as needed -maintain airway -ventilate patient -antidotes on standby Provide support and reassurance to deal with loss of sensation and mobility Provide patient teaching regarding procedure being performed and what to expect Provide life support as needed	Evaluate drug effects: -loss of sensation -loss of movement Monitor for adverse effects: -CV effects—BP changes, arrhythmias -respiratory depression -GI upset -CNS alterations -skin breakdown -anxiety, fear Monitor for drug–drug interactions as indicated for each drug Evaluate effectiveness of patient teaching program. Evaluate effectiveness of comfort and safety measures. Constantly monitor vital signs and return to normal muscular function and sensation.
PHYSICAL EXAMINATION CV: BP, P, peripheral perfusion, ECG CNS: orientation, affect, reflexes, vision Skin: color, lesions, texture, sweating Resp: R, adventitious sounds Liver function tests, plasma esterases			

FILL IN THE BLANKS
1. pain relief, analgesia, amnesia, unconsciousness
2. loss of sensation, death
3. Induction of anesthesia
4. Balanced anesthesia
5. depolarization of nerve membrane
6. central nervous system depression
7. sensation, mobility, the ability to communicate
8. skin breakdown, self-injury, biting oneself

WORD SEARCH

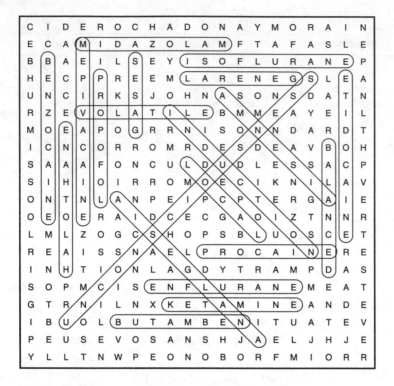

Chapter 28: Neuromuscular Junction Blocking Agents

FILL IN THE BLANKS

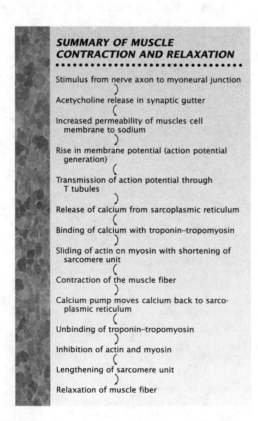

SUMMARY OF MUSCLE CONTRACTION AND RELAXATION

Stimulus from nerve axon to myoneural junction

Acetycholine release in synaptic gutter

Increased permeability of muscles cell membrane to sodium

Rise in membrane potential (action potential generation)

Transmission of action potential through T tubules

Release of calcium from sarcoplasmic reticulum

Binding of calcium with troponin–tropomyosin

Sliding of actin on myosin with shortening of sarcomere unit

Contraction of the muscle fiber

Calcium pump moves calcium back to sarcoplasmic reticulum

Unbinding of troponin–tropomyosin

Inhibition of actin and myosin

Lengthening of sarcomere unit

Relaxation of muscle fiber

CROSSWORD PUZZLE

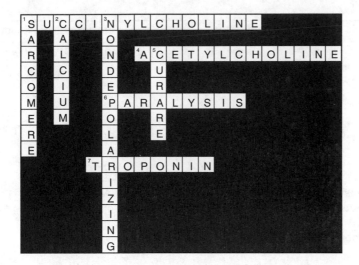

MATCHING

1. B   2. E   3. D   4. F   5. H   6. A   7. G   8. C

Chapter 29: Introduction to the Autonomic Nervous System

FILL IN THE BLANKS

COMPARISON OF THE SYMPATHETIC AND PARASYMPATHETIC NERVOUS SYSTEMS

Characteristic	Sympathetic	Parasympathetic
CNS nerve origin	Thoracic, Lumbar spinal cord	Cranium, Sacral spinal cord
Preganglionic neuron	Short axon	Long axon
Preganglionic neurotransmitter	Acetylcholine	Acetylcholine
Ganglia location	Next to spinal cord	Within or near effector organs
Postganglionic neuron	Long axon	Short axon
Postganglionic neurotransmitter	Norepinephrine	Acetylcholine
Neurotransmitter terminator	Monoamine oxidase (MAO); Catechol-D-methyltransferase (COMT)	Acetylcholinesterase
General response	Fight or flight	Rest and digest

MATCHING

1. K   2. C   3. F   4. B   5. I   6. G   7. H   8. A   9. J   10. E
11. L   12. D

FILL IN THE BLANKS

EFFECTS OF AUTONOMIC STIMULATION

Effector Site	Sympathetic Reaction	Receptor	Parasympathetic Reaction
Heart	↑ rate, contractility ↑ A-V conduction	$beta_1$	↓ Rate, ↓ A-V conduction
Blood vessels			
Skin, mucous membranes	Constriction	$alpha_1$	—
Skeletal muscle	Dilation	$beta_2$	—
Bronchial muscle	Relaxation (dilation)	$beta_2$	Constriction
GI System			
Muscle motility and tone	↓ activity	$beta_2$	↑ Activity
Sphincters	Contraction	$alpha_1$	Relaxation
Secretions	↓ secretions	$beta_2$	↑ Activity
Salivary glands	Thick secretions	$alpha_1$	Copious, watery secretions
Gallbladder	Relaxation	?	Contraction
Liver	Glyconeogenesis	$beta_2$	
Urinary bladder			
Detrusor muscle	Relaxation	$beta_2$	Contraction
Trigone muscle and sphincter	Contraction	$alpha_1$	Relaxation
Eye structures			
Iris radial muscle	Contraction (pupil dilates)	$alpha_1$	—
Iris sphincter muscle	—		Contraction (pupil constricts)
Ciliary muscle	—		contraction (lens accommodates for near vision)
Lacrimal glands	—		↑ secretions
Skin structures			
Sweat glands	↑ In sweating	Sympathetic cholinergic	—
Piloerector muscles	Contracted (goosebumps)	$alpha_1$	—
Sex organs			
Male	emission	$alpha_1$	Erection (vascular dilation)
Female	uterine relaxation	$beta_2$	—

(— means no reaction or response)

WORD SEARCH

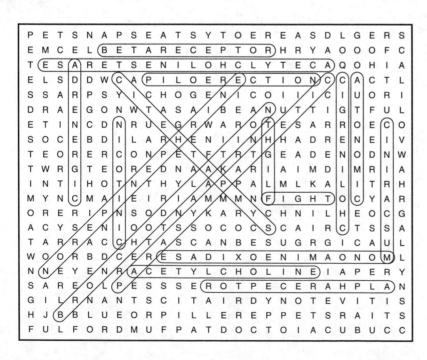

Chapter 30: Adrenergic Agents

MULTIPLE CHOICE

1. b   2. a   3. c   4. a   5. b   6. b   7. c   8. d   9. b   10. b

WORD SCRAMBLE

1. ephedrine
2. clonidine
3. dopamine
4. ritodrine
5. dobutamine
6. norepinephrine
7. metaraminol
8. phenylephrine
9. epinephrine
10. isoproterenol

FILL IN THE BLANKS

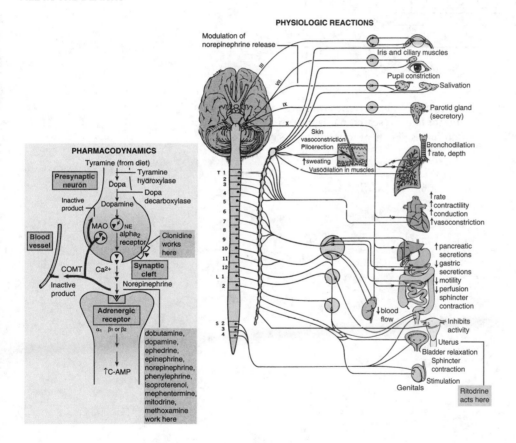

Chapter 31: Adrenergic Blocking Agents

WORD SEARCH

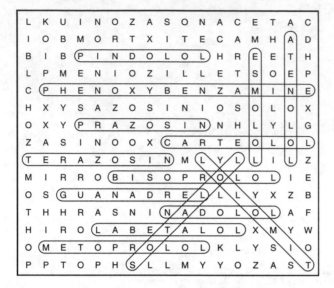

WEB EXERCISE

Go to http://www.americanheart.org, the American Heart Association website. Look up risk factors, support groups, diet, exercise, and the latest research on hypertension and other cardiovascular diseases. Print out information that is pertinent to the patient's concerns.

TRUE OR FALSE

1. F   2. T   3. F   4. T   5. T   6. F   7. T   8. T

MATCHING

1. D   2. I   3. K   4. E   5. J   6. H   7. B   8. G   9. A   10. L
11. F   12. C

Chapter 32: Cholinergic Agents

FILL IN THE BLANKS

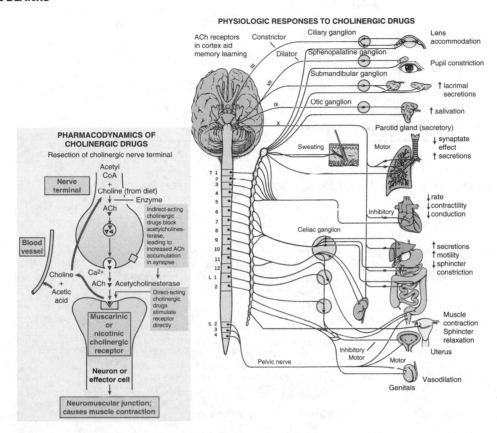

PHYSIOLOGIC RESPONSES TO CHOLINERGIC DRUGS

CROSSWORD PUZZLE

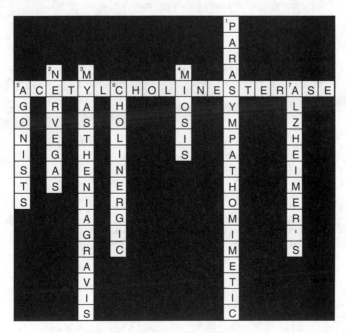

MATCHING

1. D   2. E   3. A and C   4. B   5. B   6. A and C   7. D   8. E

FILL IN THE BLANKS

1. acetylcholine
2. parasympathomimetic
3. Direct-acting
4. indirect-acting
5. Alzheimer's disease
6. Myasthenia gravis
7. nausea, vomiting, diarrhea, increased salivation
8. bradycardia, hypotension, heart block

Chapter 33: Anticholinergic Agents

FILL IN THE CHART

EFFECTS OF PARASYMPATHETIC BLOCKADE AND ASSOCIATED THERAPEUTIC USES

Psychologic Effect	Therapeutic Use
GI TRACT Smooth muscle: blocks spasms, blocks peristalsis Secretory glands; decreases acid and digestive enzyme production	Decreases motility and secretory activity in peptic ulcer, gastritis cardiospasm, pylorospasm, enteritis, diarrhea, hypertonic constipation
URINARY TRACT Decreases tone and motility in the ureters and fundus of the bladder; increases tone in the bladder sphincter	Increases bladder capacity in children with enuresis, spastic paraplegics; decreases urinary urgency and frequency in cystitis; antispasmodic in renal colic and to counteract bladder spasm caused by morphine
BILIARY TRACT Relaxes smooth muscle, antispasmodic	Relief of biliary colic; counteracts spasms caused by narcotics
BRONCHIAL MUSCLE Weakly relaxes smooth muscle	Aerosol form may be used in asthma; may counteract bronchoconstriction caused by drugs
CARDIOVASCULAR SYSTEM Increases heart rate (may decrease heart rate at very low doses); causes local vasodilation and flushing	Counteracts bradycardia caused by vagal stimulation, carotid sinus syndrome, surgical procedures; used to overcome heart blocks following MI; used to counteract hypotension caused by cholinergic drugs.
OCULAR EFFECTS Pupil dilation, cyclopegia	Allows ophthalmological examination of the retina, optic disk; relaxes ocular muscles and decreases irritation in iridocyclitis, choroiditis
SECRETIONS Reduces sweating, salivation, respiratory tract secretions	Preoperatively before inhalation anesthesia; reduces nasal secretions in rhinitis, hay fever; may be used to reduce excessive sweating in hyperhidrosis
CNS Decreases extrapyramidal motor activity Atropine may cause excessive stimulation, psychosis, delirium, disorientation Scopolamine causes depression, drowsiness	Decreases tremor in parkinsonism; helps to prevent motion sickness; scopolamine may be in OTC sleep aids

PATIENT TEACHING CHECKLIST

DICYCLOMINE

Parasympathetic blockers or anticholinergics block or stop the actions of a group of nerves that are part of the sympathetic nervous system. This drug may decrease the activity of your gastrointestinal (GI) tract, dilate your pupils, or increase your heart rate.

Common effects of these drugs include:

- Dry mouth, difficulty swallowing—Frequent mouth care will help to remove dried secretions and keep the mouth fresh; sucking on sugarless candies will help to keep the mouth moist; taking lots of fluids with meals (unless you are on a fluid restriction) will help aid swallowing.
- Blurring vision, sensitivity to light—If your vision is blurred, avoid driving, operating hazardous machinery, or doing close work that requires attention to details until vision returns to normal; dark glasses will help to protect your eyes from the light.
- Retention of urine—Taking the drug just after you have emptied your bladder will help; moderate your fluid intake when the drug's effects are the highest; if possible, take the drug before bed when this effect will not be a problem.
- Constipation—Include fluid and roughage in your diet; follow any bowel regimen that you may have; monitor your bowel movements so that appropriate laxatives can be taken if necessary.
- Flushing, intolerance to heat, decreased sweating—This drug blocks sweating, which is your body's way of cooling off; avoid extremes of temperature; dress coolly; on very warm days, avoid exercise as much as possible.

Report any of the following to your health care provider: eye pain, skin rash, fever, rapid heart beat, chest pain, difficulty breathing, agitation or mood changes, impotence (a dosage adjustment may help alleviate this problem).

Avoid the use of over-the-counter (OTC) medications, especially for sleep and nasal congestion; avoid antihistamines, diet pills, cold capsules. These drugs may contain similar drugs that could cause a severe reaction. Consult with your health care provider if you believe that you need medication for symptomatic relief.

Tell any doctor, nurse, or other health care provider that you are taking these drugs.

Keep this drug, and all medications, out of the reach of children. Do not share these drugs with other people.

Specific information to keep in mind with this anticholinergic drug:

- Make sure you empty your bladder before taking the drug.
- Return for your follow-up visit in 4 weeks for evaluation for increasing the dosage.

FILL IN THE BLANKS

1. acetylcholine
2. parasympatholytic
3. increase, decrease
4. sweating
5. Cyclopegia
6. mydriatic
7. Atropine
8. dry mouth, difficulty swallowing

CROSSWORD PUZZLE

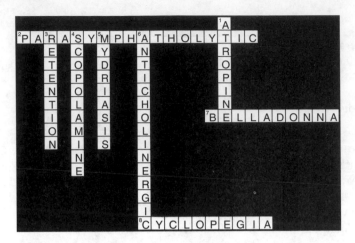

Chapter 34: Introduction to the Endocrine System

FILL IN THE BLANKS

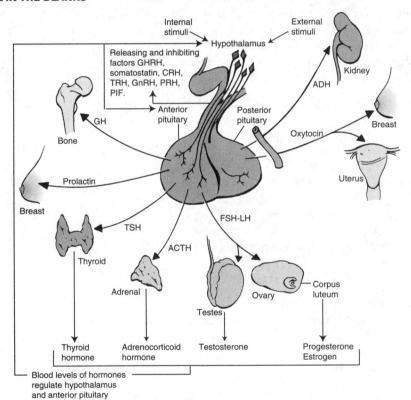

LISTING

1. are produced in very small amounts
2. are secreted directly into the bloodstream
3. travel through the blood to specific receptor sites throughout the body
4. act to increase or decrease the normal metabolic processes of cells when they react with their specific receptor sites
5. are immediately broken down

MATCHING

1. D   2. H   3. F   4. A   5. G   6. C   7. E   8. B

WORD SCRAMBLE

1. pituitary gland
2. diurnal rhythm
3. releasing factors
4. insulin
5. hypothalamus
6. negative feedback
7. hormones
8. posterior pituitary
9. pancreas
10. hypothalamic–pituitary axis

Chapter 35: Hypothalamic and Pituitary Agents

MATCHING

1. F   2. G   3. B   4. A   5. D   6. E   7. C

WEB EXERCISE

Go to http://www.aace.com, the American Association of Clinical Endocrinologists home page. Check on Publications, Clinical Guidelines, and Guidelines for growth hormone use in adults and children. Print out appropriate pages to prepare handouts or a poster for your presentation.

MATCHING

1. C   2. E   3. G   4. A   5. D   6. H   7. B   8. F

WORD SEARCH

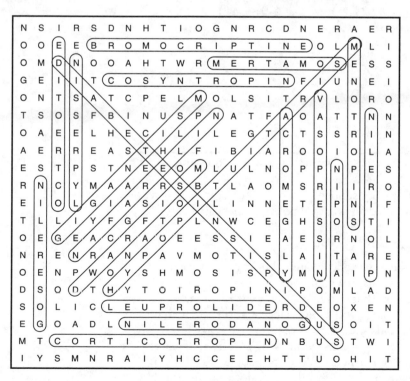

Chapter 36: Adrenocortical Agents

WORD SCRAMBLE

1. prednisone
2. triamcinolone
3. betamethasone
4. hydrocortisone
5. budesonide
6. flunisolide
7. cortisone
8. dexamethasone

CROSSWORD PUZZLE

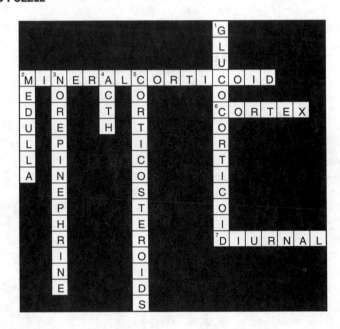

TRUE OR FALSE

1. F   2. F   3. F   4. T   5. T   6. F   7. F   8. T   9. T   10. T

PATIENT TEACHING CHECKLIST

CORTICOSTEROIDS

Corticosteroids are similar to steroids produced naturally in your body and affect a number of bodily functions.

You should never stop taking your drug suddenly. If your prescription is low, or you are unable to take the medication for any reason, notify your health care provider.

Some of the following adverse effects may occur:

- Increased appetite—This may be a welcome change, but if you notice a continual weight gain, you may want to watch your calories. This drug should ease the cramping and pain that you have been experiencing.
- Restlessness, trouble sleeping—Some people experience elation and a feeling of new energy; frequent rest periods should be taken.
- Increased susceptibility to infection—Because your body's normal defenses will be decreased, you should avoid crowded places or people with known infections. If you notice any signs of illness or infection, notify your health

care provider at once. You should avoid crowded areas and be particularly careful to avoid injury.

If you are taking this drug for a prolonged period of time, limit your intake of salt and salted products and add proteins to your diet.

Avoid the use of any over-the-counter (OTC) medication without first checking with your health care provider. Several of these medications can interfere with the effectiveness of this drug.

Tell any doctor, nurse, or other health care provider that you are taking this drug.

Because this drug affects your body's natural defenses, you will need special care during any stressful situations. You may want to wear or carry a medical-alert tag showing that you are on this medication. This tag alerts any medical personnel taking care of you in an emergency that you are taking this drug.

Report any of the following to your health care provider: sudden weight gain; fever or sore throat; black, tarry stools; swelling of the hands or feet; any signs of infection; easy bruising.

It is important to have regular medical follow-up. If you are being tapered from this drug, notify your health care provider if any of the following occur: fatigue; nausea, vomiting; diarrhea; weight loss; weakness; dizziness.

Keep this drug, and all medications, out of the reach of children. Do not give this medication to anyone else or take any similar medication that has not been prescribed for you.

Chapter 37: Thyroid and Parathyroid Agents

PATIENT TEACHING CHECKLIST

THYROID HORMONE

A hormone is designed to replace the thyroid hormone that your body is not able to produce. The thyroid hormone is responsible for regulating your body's metabolism, or the speed with which your body's cells burn energy. Because of this action of the thyroid hormone, it affects many body systems. It is very important that you take this medication only as prescribed.

Never stop taking this drug without consulting with your health care provider. The drug is used to replace an important hormone and will probably have to be taken for life. Stopping the medication can lead to serious problems.

This drug usually causes no adverse effects. You may notice a slight skin rash or hair loss in the first few months of therapy. You should notice that the signs and symptoms of your thyroid deficiency will disappear and you will feel "back to normal."

Report any of the following to your health care provider: chest pain, difficulty breathing, sore throat, fever, chills, weight gain, sleeplessness, nervousness, unusual sweating, or intolerance to heat.

Avoid the use of any over-the-counter (OCT) medications without first checking with your health care provider. Several of these medications can interfere with the effectiveness of this drug.

Tell any doctor, nurse, or other health care provider that you are taking this drug. You may want to wear or carry a medical-alert tag showing that you are on this medication. This would alert any medical personnel taking care of you in an emergency that you are taking this drug.

When you are taking this drug, it is important to have regular medical follow-up, including blood tests to check the activity of your thyroid gland, to evaluate your response to the drug and any possible underlying problems.

Keep this drug, and all medications, out of the reach of children. Do not give this medication to anyone else or take any similar medication that has not been prescribed for you.

You should start feeling like your old self again soon. Your energy should return and you should regain interest in things. The dosage of your thyroid hormone may need to be adjusted. It is very important that you keep return appointments, which will include blood tests, so that the appropriate dosage can be determined. If you have any questions, please feel free to call the office at 555-5555 and ask to speak to Nurse Jones.

MULTIPLE CHOICE

1. a   2. c   3. c   4. d   5. b   6. d

MATCHING

1. E   2. A   3. F   4. B   5. J   6. C   7. H   8. D   9. G   10. I

WORD SCRAMBLE

1. calcitonin
2. thyroxine
3. cretinism
4. bisphosphonates
5. parathormone
6. iodine
7. osteoporosis
8. hyperthyroidism
9. myxedema
10. liothyronine

Chapter 38: Antidiabetic Agents

WORD SEARCH

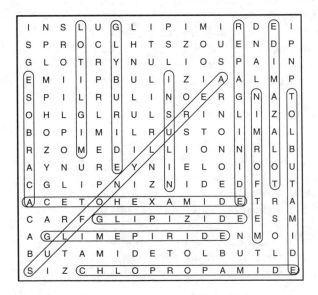

WEB EXERCISE

Go to http://www.diabetes.org, the American Diabetes Association (ADA) website. Click "Type 2 Diabetes" to get information about the disease. Click "Medical Information" to get information about the specific drugs that J. L. might be taking. Click "Meal Planning" to get nutrition information as well as recipes that J. L. or his wife might like to review. If they seem interested in support groups, enter their ZIP code to find the local ADA chapter and pertinent support. Print out anything that would be useful in preparing a teaching program for this patient.

NURSING CARE PLAN

Insulin

Assessment	Nursing Diagnoses	Implementation	Evaluation
HISTORY Allergies to any insulins	Improved nutrition related to metabolic effect	Administer SC and rotate sites	Evaluate drug effects: return of glucose levels to normal.
	Altered sensory perception related to effects on glucose levels	Store in cool place away from light	Monitor for adverse effects: hypoglycemia injection site reaction.
	Risk for infection related to injections and disease process	Use caution when mixing types	Monitor for drug-drug interactions: delayed recovery from hypo- glycemic episodes with propranolol (*Inderal*).
	Impaired coping related to diagnosis and injections	Monitor blood glucose to adjust dosage as needed	Evaluate effectiveness of patient teaching pro- gram.
	Deficient knowledge regarding drug therapy	Monitor during times of stress and trauma and adjust dosage	Evaluate effectiveness of comfort and safety measures.
		Provide support and reas- surance to deal with drug injections and life- time need	
		Provide patient teaching regarding drug name, dosage, adverse effects, precautions, warning signs to report, and proper administration technique	
PHYSICAL EXAMINATION Neurological: orientation, reflexes Skin: color, lesions CV: P, cardiac ausculta- tion, BP Respiratory: R, adventi- tious sounds Lab tests: urinalysis, blood glucose			

FILL IN THE BLANKS

1. diabetes mellitus
2. insulin, glucagon, somatostatin
3. glycogen, lipids, proteins
4. glycosuria
5. polyphagia
6. Polydipsia
7. ketosis
8. diet, exercise
9. sulfonylureas
10. metformin

Chapter 39: Introduction to the Reproductive System

FILL IN THE BLANKS

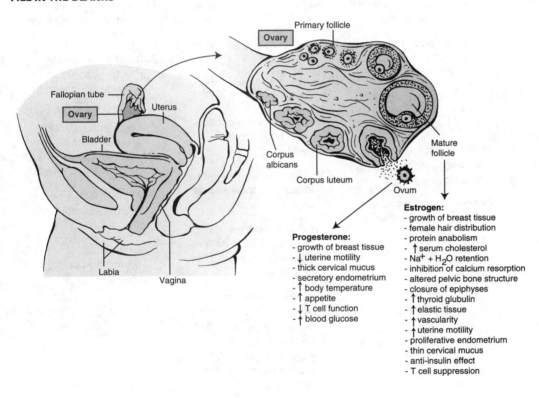

Progesterone:
- growth of breast tissue
- ↓ uterine motility
- thick cervical mucus
- secretory endometrium
- ↑ body temperature
- ↑ appetite
- ↓ T cell function
- ↑ blood glucose

Estrogen:
- growth of breast tissue
- female hair distribution
- protein anabolism
- ↑ serum cholesterol
- Na^+ + H_2O retention
- inhibition of calcium resorption
- altered pelvic bone structure
- closure of epiphyses
- ↑ thyroid glubulin
- ↑ elastic tissue
- ↑ vascularity
- ↑ uterine motility
- proliferative endometrium
- thin cervical mucus
- anti-insulin effect
- T cell suppression

FILL IN THE BLANKS

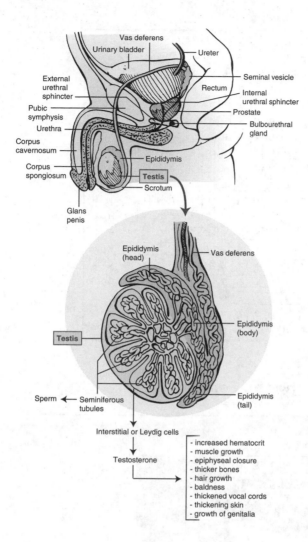

FILL IN THE BLANKS

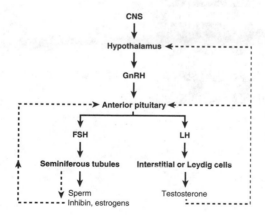

WORD SEARCH

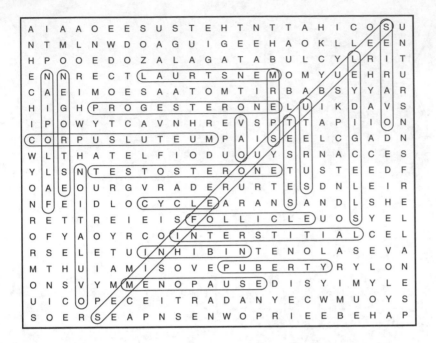

Chapter 40: Drugs Affecting the Female Reproductive System

CROSSWORD PUZZLE

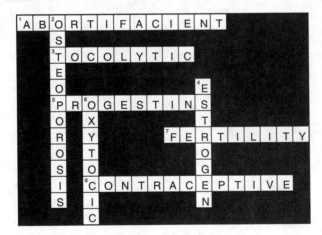

MULTIPLE CHOICE

1. d   2. a   3. b   4. b   5. b   6. c

WORD SCRAMBLE

1. toremifene
2. estradiol
3. estrone
4. raloxifene
5. dienestrol
6. estropipate
7. diethylstilbestrol
8. chlorotrianisene

FILL IN THE BLANKS

1. oxytocics
2. tocolytics
3. osteoporosis, hot flashes, coronary artery disease
4. thrombi, emboli
5. Raloxifene
6. progestin
7. fertility drugs
8. abortifacients

Chapter 41: Drugs Affecting the Male Reproductive System

TRUE OR FALSE

1. T   2. F   3. T   4. T   5. F   6. F   7. T   8. T   9. F   10. F

MATCHING

1. D   2. E   3. A   4. G   5. C   6. H   7. B   8. F

FILL IN THE BLANKS

1. Androgenic
2. Anabolic
3. Testosterone
4. anemias
5. Erectile penile dysfunction
6. prostaglandin, injected
7. Sildenafil
8. sexual stimulation

WORD SCRAMBLE

1. hirsutism
2. hypogonadism
3. anabolic
4. sildenafil
5. androgens
6. erectile dysfunction
7. testosterone
8. alprostadil
9. nandrolone
10. danazol

Chapter 42: Introduction to the Cardiovascular System

FILL IN THE BLANKS

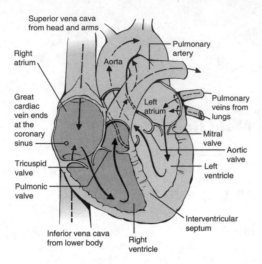

Superior vena cava
from head and arms

Right
atrium

Aorta

Pulmonary
artery

Great
cardiac
vein ends
at the
coronary
sinus

Left
atrium

Pulmonary
veins from
lungs

Mitral
valve

Aortic
valve

Tricuspid
valve

Left
ventricle

Pulmonic
valve

Interventricular
septum

Inferior vena cava
from lower body

Right
ventricle

DEFINITIONS

1. troponin: chemical in heart muscle that prevents actin and myosin from reacting, leading to muscle relaxation; inactivated by calcium during muscle stimulation to allow actin and myosin to react, causing muscle contraction
2. actin: thin filament that makes up a sarcomere or muscle unit
3. myosin: thick filament with projections that makes up a sarcomere or muscle unit
4. arrhythmia: a disruption in cardiac rate or rhythm
5. Starling's law of the heart: addresses the contractile properties of the heart; the more the muscle is stretched, the stronger it will react until stretched to a point at which it will not react at all
6. fibrillation: rapid, irregular stimulation of the cardiac muscle resulting in lack of pumping activity
7. capillary: small vessel made up of loosely connected endothelial cells that connect arteries to veins
8. resistance system: the arteries; the muscles of the arteries provide resistance to the flow of blood, leading to control of blood pressure

MATCHING

1. H   2. C   3. F   4. E   5. D   6. L   7. J   8. A   9. K   10. G
11. I   12. B

CROSSWORD PUZZLE

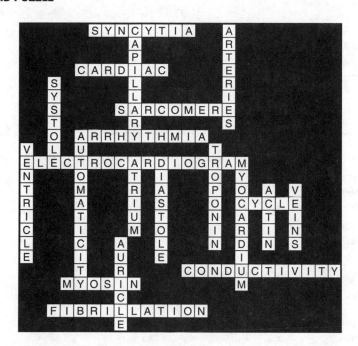

Chapter 43: Drugs Affecting Blood Pressure

MATCHING

1. B   2. A   3. E   4. B   5. D   6. D   7. A   8. B   9. C   10. D

11. A   12. C

WORD SEARCH

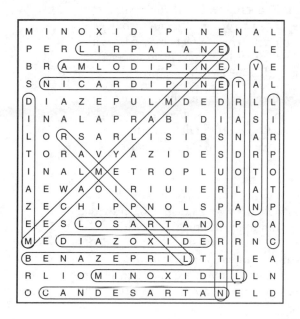

TRUE OR FALSE

1. F   2. T   3. F   4. F   5. T   6. F   7. T   8. T   9. F   10. T

MATCHING

1. D   2. I   3. F   4. C   5. J   6. A   7. G   8. E   9. H   10. B

Chapter 44: Cardiotonic Agents

PATIENT TEACHING CHECKLIST

DIGOXIN

Digoxin is a digitalis preparation. Digitalis has many helpful effects on the heart. It helps it to beat more slowly and efficiently. These effects lead to better circulation and should help to reduce the swelling in your ankles or legs and should increase the amount of urine that you produce every day. Digoxin is a powerful drug and must be taken *exactly* as prescribed. It is important to have regular medical checkups to ensure that the dosage of the drug is correct for you and to be sure that it is having the desired effect on your heart.

Do not stop taking this drug without consulting your health care provider. Never skip doses and never try to "catch up" on any missed doses; serious adverse effects could occur.

You should learn to take your own pulse. You should take your pulse each morning before engaging in any activity. Your normal pulse rate is 82.

You should monitor your weight fairly closely. Weigh yourself every other day at the same time of the day and wearing the same amount of clothing. Record your weight on your calendar for easy reference. If you gain or lose 3 or more pounds in one day, it may indicate a problem with your drug. Consult your health care provider. Your weight today is 148 pounds, fully clothed with shoes.

Common effects of these drugs include:

- Dizziness, drowsiness, headache—Avoid driving or performing hazardous tasks or delicate tasks that require concentration if these occur. Consult your health care provider for an appropriate analgesic if the headache is a problem.
- Nausea, GI upset, loss of appetite—Small, frequent meals may help; monitor your weight loss and if it becomes severe, consult your health care provider.
- Vision changes, "yellow" halos around objects—These effects may pass with time. Take extra care in your activities for the first few days. If these reactions do not go away after 3 to 4 days, consult with your health care provider.

Report any of the following to your health care provider: unusually slow or irregular pulse; rapid weight gain; "yellow vision"; unusual tiredness or weakness; skin rash or hives; swelling of the ankles, legs, or fingers; difficulty breathing.

Tell any doctor, nurse, dentist, or other health care provider that you are taking this drug.

Keep this drug, and all medications, out of the reach of children.

Avoid the use of over-the-counter (OTC) medications when you are on this drug. If you feel that you need one of these, consult with your health care provider for the best choice. Many of these drugs may contain ingredients that could interfere with your digoxin.

It might be helpful to wear or carry a medical-alert tag to alert any medical personnel who might take care of you in an emergency that you are taking this drug.

Regular medical follow-up is important to evaluate the actions of the drug and to adjust the dosage if necessary.

Specifics related to your situation:

- Be very careful the first few days in Florida. The change in temperatures may tend to make you light headed and dizzy.
- Contact your health care provider in Florida as soon as possible to alert him to your new prescription.

CROSSWORD PUZZLE

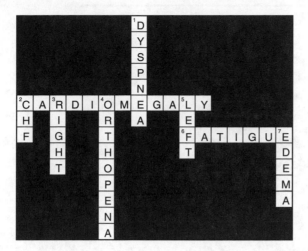

WEB EXERCISE

Go to the American Heart Association home page at http://www.americanheart.org. Select "Your Heart." Now select "Diseases and Conditions." Then select "Congestive Heart Failure." Print out pertinent information that might be useful for J.D. Return to the home page and enter your ZIP code, then print out information on support groups and help in your specific area.

WORD SCRAMBLE

1. dyspnea
2. milrinone
3. nocturia
4. orthopnea
5. tachypnea
6. congestive heart failure
7. digoxin
8. hemoptysis
9. cardiomyopathy
10. immune fab

Chapter 45: Antiarrhythmic Agents

FILL IN THE BLANKS

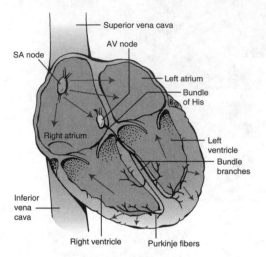

MATCHING

1. B, D   2. A, F   3. C, E

WORD SCRAMBLE

1. amiodarone
2. esmolol
3. bretylium
4. verapamil
5. procainamide
6. propranolol
7. flecainide
8. digoxin

FILL IN THE BLANKS

1. tachycardias, bradycardias
2. cardiac output
3. action potential
4. CAST study
5. automaticity
6. β-receptor
7. digoxin
8. lidocaine

Chapter 46: Antianginal Agents

MATCHING

1. C   2. F   3. E   4. G   5. A   6. B   7. D   8. H

TRUE OR FALSE

1. F   2. T   3. F   4. T   5. F   6. F   7. T   8. T

CROSSWORD PUZZLE

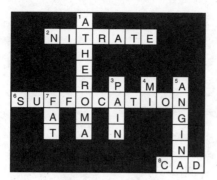

WORD SEARCH

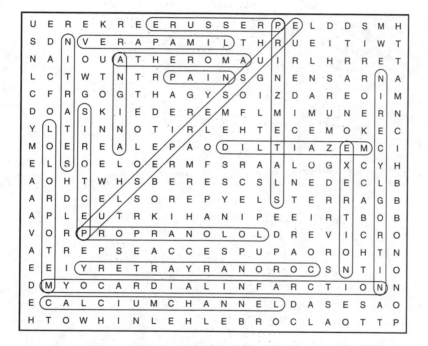

Chapter 47: Lipid-Lowering Agents

WEB EXERCISE

Go to the American Heart Association home page at http://www.americanheart.org. Click on "Warning Signs," then "Risk Assessment" for a survey of risk factors. Return to the home page. Click on "Diseases and Conditions," then "Cholesterol" for diet and drug guidelines and print out useful material.

LISTING

1. Genetic predispositions
2. Age
3. Gender
4. Gout—M
5. Cigarette smoking—M
6. Sedentary lifestyle—M
7. High stress levels—M
8. Hypertension—M
9. Obesity—M
10. Diabetes—M

FILL IN THE BLANKS

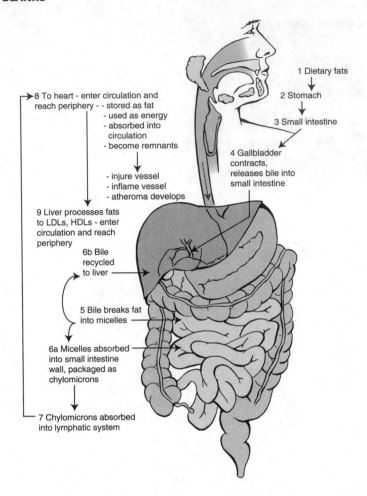

1 Dietary fats

2 Stomach

3 Small intestine

4 Gallbladder contracts, releases bile into small intestine

8 To heart - enter circulation and reach periphery - - stored as fat
- used as energy
- absorbed into circulation
- become remnants

- injure vessel
- inflame vessel
- atheroma develops

9 Liver processes fats to LDLs, HDLs - enter circulation and reach periphery

6b Bile recycled to liver

5 Bile breaks fat into micelles

6a Micelles absorbed into small intestine wall, packaged as chylomicrons

7 Chylomicrons absorbed into lymphatic system

WORD SCRAMBLE

1. cholesterol
2. clofibrate
3. niacin
4. hyperlipidemia
5. colestipol
6. atorvastatin
7. gemfibrozil
8. bile acids
9. lipoprotein
10. lovastatin

Chapter 48: Drugs Affecting Blood Coagulation

TRUE OR FALSE

1. T   2. F   3. T   4. F   5. T   6. F   7. T   8. F   9. F   10. T

FILL IN THE BLANKS

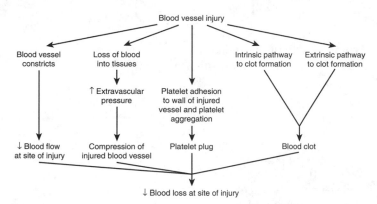

PATIENT TEACHING CHECKLIST

COUMADIN

An anticoagulant works to slow the normal blood clotting processes in the body. In this way, it can prevent harmful blood clots from forming. This type of drug is often called a "blood thinner." It cannot dissolve any blood clots that have already formed. Your anticoagulant has been prescribed because ——————.

Never change any medication that you are taking—adding or stopping another drug—without consulting with your health care provider. Many other drugs affect the way that your anticoagulant works; starting or stopping another drug can cause excessive bleeding or interfere with the desired effects of the drug.

Your drug should be taken once a day. The best time of day to take your drug is in the morning.

Common effects of these drugs include:

- Stomach bloating, cramps—This often passes with time; consult your health care provider if this persists or becomes too uncomfortable.
- Loss of hair, skin rash—This can be very frustrating. You may wish to discuss this with your health care provider.
- Orange-yellow discoloration of the urine—This can be frightening, but may just be an effect of the drug. If you are concerned that this might be blood, simply add vinegar to your urine. The color should disappear. If the color does not disappear, it may be caused by blood and you should contact your health care provider.

Report any of the following to your health care provider: unusual bleeding (eg, when brushing your teeth); excessive bleeding from an injury; excessive bruising; black or tarry stools; cloudy or dark urine; sore throat, fever, chills; severe headache or dizziness.

Tell any doctor, nurse, or other health care provider that you are taking this drug. You should carry or wear a medical-alert tag stating that you are on this drug. This will alert emergency medical personnel that you are at increased risk for bleeding.

It is important to avoid situations in which you could be easily injured—for example, contact sports, using a straight razor.

Keep this drug, and all medications, out of the reach of children.

Avoid the use of over-the-counter (OTC) medications when you are on this drug. If you feel that you need one of these, consult with your health care provider for the best choice. Many of these drugs may interfere with your anticoagulant.

You will need to have regular, periodic blood tests when you are on this drug.

This is very important for monitoring the effects of the drug on your body and adjusting your dosage as needed.

Specifics related to your situation:

- Use extra care to prevent injury when playing with the children.
- If you change your diet or cannot take your medication, consult with your health care provider.

CROSSWORD PUZZLE

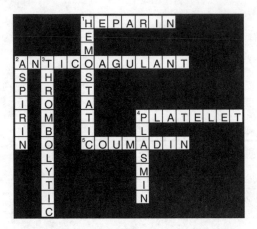

Chapter 49: Drugs Used to Treat Anemias

FILL IN THE BLANKS

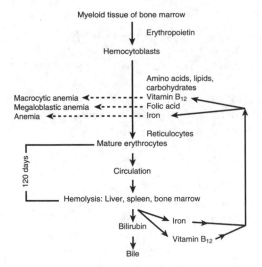

MULTIPLE CHOICE

1. a   2. c   3. b   4. d   5. a   6. c

CROSSWORD PUZZLE

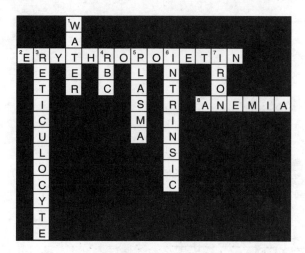

WORD SCRAMBLE

1. erythrocytes
2. plasma
3. megaloblastic
4. pernicious
5. epoetin
6. folic acid
7. anemia
8. erythropoiesis
9. reticulocyte
10. deficiency

Chapter 50: Introduction to the Kidney and the Urinary Tract

FILL IN THE BLANKS

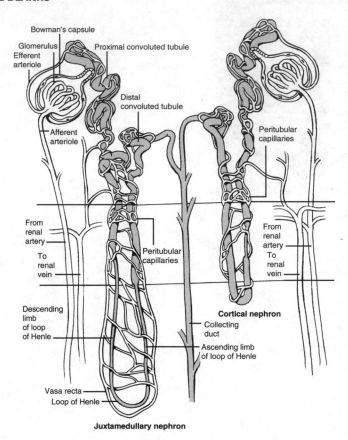

Bowman's capsule
Glomerulus
Efferent arteriole
Proximal convoluted tubule
Distal convoluted tubule
Afferent arteriole
Peritubular capillaries
From renal artery
To renal vein
Peritubular capillaries
From renal artery
To renal vein
Descending limb of loop of Henle
Cortical nephron
Collecting duct
Ascending limb of loop of Henle
Vasa recta
Loop of Henle
Juxtamedullary nephron

WORD SCRAMBLE

1. glomerulus
2. filtration
3. secretion
4. aldosterone
5. reabsorption
6. tubule
7. renin
8. prostate

FILL IN THE BLANKS

1. 25%
2. nephron, Bowman's capsule, loop of Henle, collecting duct
3. glomerular filtration, tubular secretion, tubular reabsorption
4. aldosterone
5. concentration, dilution
6. aldosterone
7. Vitamin D
8. renin

CROSSWORD PUZZLE

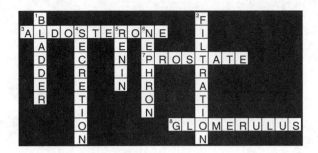

Chapter 51: Diuretic Agents

WORD SEARCH

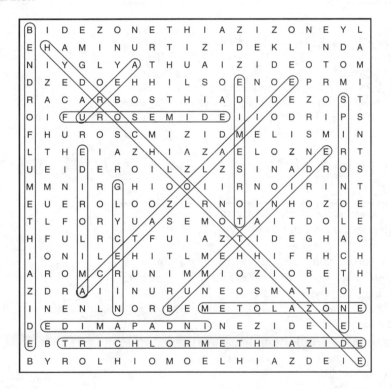

DEFINITIONS

1. edema: movement of fluid into the interstitial spaces; occurs when the balance between osmotic pull (from plasma proteins) and hydrostatic push (from blood pressure) is upset
2. fluid rebound: reflex reaction of the body to the loss of fluid or sodium; hypothalamus causes the release of ADH, which retains water, and stress related to fluid loss combines with decreased blood flow to the kidneys to activate the renin–angiotensin system, leading to further water and sodium retention
3. thiazide: a type of diuretic acting in the renal tubule to block the chloride pump, which prevents the reabsorption of sodium and chloride, leading to a loss of sodium and water in the urine
4. hypokalemia: low potassium in the blood; often occurs after diuretic use; characterized by weakness, muscle cramps, trembling, nausea, vomiting, diarrhea, and cardiac arrhythmias
5. high-ceiling diuretics: powerful diuretics that work in the loop of Henle to inhibit the reabsorption of sodium and chloride, leading to a sodium-rich diuresis
6. alkalosis: state of not having enough acid to maintain normal homeostatic processes; seen with loop diuretics, which cause the loss of bicarbonate in the urine

7. hyperaldosteronism: excessive output of aldosterone from the adrenal gland, leading to increased sodium and water retention and loss of potassium

8. osmotic pull: drawing force of large molecules on water, pulling it into the tubule or capillary; essential for maintaining normal fluid balance within the body; used to draw out excess fluid into the vascular system or the renal tubule

MATCHING

1. A   2. E   3. C   4. B   5. B   6. A   7. D   8. B   9. D   10. C

MULTIPLE CHOICE

1. c   2. d   3. b   4. d   5. a   6. d   7. b   8. c

Chapter 52: Drugs Affecting the Urinary Tract and Bladder

WEB EXERCISE

Using your web browser, go to http://www.pslgroup.com/ENLARGPROST.HTM. On the home page, click on "Enlarged Prostate Information," then click on "The Prostate Gland" to get information about the location and function of the gland and problems that occur. Print this information, if appropriate. Go back to "Enlarged Prostate Information," click on "Treatment," then select pertinent facts. Finally, return to the home page and scan the other buttons you can click for additional material (eg, PSA levels, use of the TUNA approach) that might be helpful to your patient.

PATIENT TEACHING CHECKLIST

URINARY TRACT ANTI-INFECTIVES

A urinary tract anti-infective works to treat urinary tract infections by destroying bacteria and by helping to produce an environment that is not conducive to bacteria growth.

If this drug causes stomach upset, it can be taken with food. It is important to avoid foods that alkalinize the urine—for example, citrus fruits and milk—because they decrease the effectiveness of the drug. Cranberry juice is one juice that can be used. Fluids should be pushed as much as possible (8 to 10 glasses of water a day) to help treat the infection.

Avoid the use of any over-the-counter (OTC) medication that might contain sodium bicarbonate (eg, antacids, baking soda). If you question the use of any OTC drug, check with your health care provider.

Take the full course of your prescription. Do not use this drug to self-treat any other infection.

Common effects of this drug that you should be aware of include:

- Stomach upset, nausea—Taking the drug with food may help; small, frequent meals may also help.
- Painful urination—If this occurs, report it to your health care provider. A dosage adjustment may be needed.

There are several other activities that could help to decrease urinary tract infections and should be considered when you are on this drug as well as at other times:

- Avoid bubble baths
- Women should always wipe from front to back, never from back to front.
- Void whenever you feel the urge; try not to wait.
- Always try to void after sexual intercourse to flush the urethra.

Report any of the following to your health care provider: skin rash or itching, severe gastrointestinal (GI) upset, GI upset that prevents adequate fluid intake, very painful urination, pregnancy.

Tell any doctor, nurse, or other health care provider that you are taking this drug.

Keep this drug, and all medications, out of the reach of children.

TRUE OR FALSE

1. T   2. F   3. F   4. T   5. F   6. T   7. F   8. T

WORD SCRAMBLE

1. dysuria
2. nocturia
3. urgency
4. frequency
5. cystitis
6. doxazosin
7. oxybutynin
8. acidification
9. antispasmodics
10. pyelonephritis

Chapter 53: Introduction to the Respiratory System

FILL IN THE BLANKS

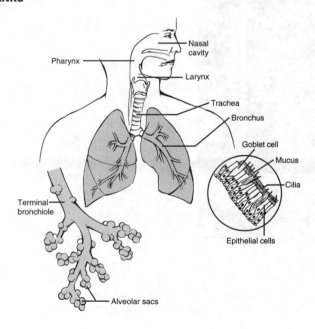

MATCHING

1. K   2. D   3. B   4. J   5. E   6. A   7. C   8. G   9. L   10. F
11. I   12. H

MULTIPLE CHOICE

1. a   2. c   3. d   4. c   5. d   6. b   7. a   8. b

WORD SEARCH

```
N I U T L T U C T O Y T H I S E D R A T S
T S R RESPIRATION B S A A D N A
E E S U C L R U A N P F Y I L O E V L A H
W T I L RHINITIS L O A O E N S I T
L N N R E R O A N E O L N A S N D R I N L
D A U H T U N I O L A I E A T D U E N O A
C T S O T E I L R I U H E I E T L P U M U
R C E S O B R I H A C F LOWER P S U S O
E A S R E U E C M A D ASTHMA U I E O
D F L A R Y N X R P T D H E G A A L T N D
I R R Y Z O P T O I N E U H U L B Y I P C
C U O N R S E COMMONCOLD U S I R
R S M B V O I N SNEEZE C R I E S T A
O M A PULMONARY A N D E T R E I D
H N I L I N S L A N D R D N O M S A S E P
```

Chapter 54: Drugs Acting on the Upper Respiratory Tract

CROSSWORD PUZZLE

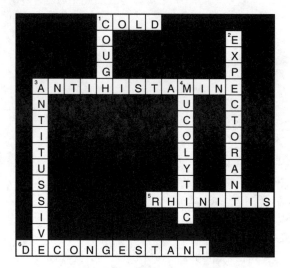

WEB EXERCISE

Using your web browser, go to http://www.nlm.nih.gov/medlineplus/healthtopics.html. Select "A," then "Allergy." Print out pertinent pages to prepare a teaching program for R. W.

WORD SCRAMBLE

1. clemastine
2. dextromethorphan
3. ephedrine
4. tetrahydrozoline
5. pseudoephedrine
6. budesonide
7. fluticasone
8. astemizole

MATCHING

1. E   2. G   3. H   4. J   5. I   6. A   7. F   8. C   9. B   10. D

Chapter 55: Drugs Used to Treat Obstructive Pulmonary Disorders

TRUE OR FALSE

1. F   2. T   3. T   4. F   5. F   6. F   7. T   8. T

WEB EXERCISE

Using your web browser, go to http://www.lungusa.org. Select "Diseases A to Z" from the column on the left, then go to "Tuberculosis." Scroll down through the disease, symptoms, risks, diagnosis, and treatments. Return to the home page. Select "Research." Return to the home page. At the bottom of the page you can select "Find Another Association Here" by entering a ZIP code.

WORD SEARCH

```
B  O  X  T  R  I  P  H  Y  L  L  I  N  E  X  E
R  I  N  E  O  P  H  Y  L  L  I  N  E  E  P  R
E  A  M  I  N  R  B  E  R  A  C  T  A  N  T  S
N  O  M  I  N  A  O  Z  I  L  E  U  T  O  N  T
I  N  E  I  S  T  H  Y  P  B  E  R  A  C  Y  S
L  I  N  E  N  R  O  P  H  U  T  A  L  I  L  A
L  P  H  I  S  O  P  R  O  T  E  R  E  N  O  L
Y  M  I  N  O  P  P  I  N  E  X  C  A  R  M  U
F  I  N  E  P  I  P  H  Y  R  I  S  T  O  O  K
I  N  E  Y  Z  U  L  I  Y  O  P  H  Y  L  R  R
X  O  O  H  Y  M  I  N  E  L  U  K  A  S  C  I
O  O  L  I  R  E  C  S  O  F  L  O  C  H  E  F
T  P  H  Y  L  L  C  A  F  F  E  I  N  E  X  A
N  E  D  O  C  R  O  M  I  L  X  O  N  E  A  Z
E  Z  A  F  L  U  N  I  S  O  L  I  D  E  N  E
P  I  R  B  U  T  E  R  O  L  I  O  N  P  H  Y
```

WORD SCRAMBLE

1. theophylline
2. albuterol
3. epinephrine
4. salmeterol
5. ipratropium
6. budesonide
7. zafirlukast
8. zileuton
9. beractant
10. poractant

Chapter 56: Introduction to the Gastrointestinal System

FILL IN THE BLANKS

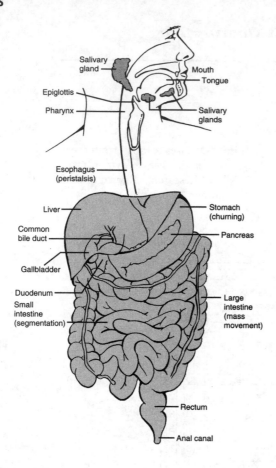

- Salivary gland
- Mouth
- Tongue
- Epiglottis
- Pharynx
- Salivary glands
- Esophagus (peristalsis)
- Liver
- Stomach (churning)
- Common bile duct
- Pancreas
- Gallbladder
- Duodenum
- Small intestine (segmentation)
- Large intestine (mass movement)
- Rectum
- Anal canal

MATCHING

1. F   2. C   3. G   4. H   5. B   6. A   7. E   8. D   9. J   10. I

FILL IN THE BLANKS

1. digestion, absorption
2. acid, mucous
3. nerve plexus
4. sympathetic, parasympathetic
5. local reflexes
6. constipation, diarrhea
7. medulla
8. chemoreceptor trigger zone (CTZ)

WORD SEARCH

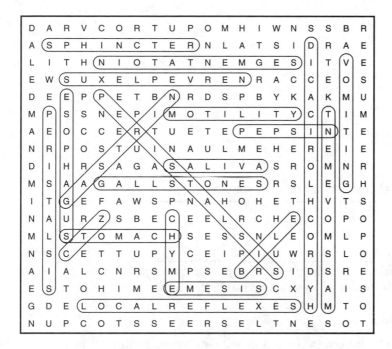

Chapter 57: Drugs Affecting Gastrointestinal Secretions

WEB EXERCISE

Using your web browser, go to http://www.nlm.nih.gov/medlineplus/healthtopics.html. Select "D," then "Digestive Diseases." Choose several different complaints and using the information presented for each one, prepare a teaching session, including the following elements: causes, life style changes, decrease occurrence, treatment, and medical follow-up.

CROSSWORD PUZZLE

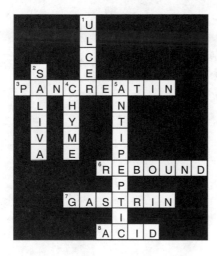

MATCHING

1. E   2. C   3. D   4. A   5. F   6. B   7. B   8. F   9. C   10. A

WORD SCRAMBLE

1. sucralfate
2. pancreatin
3. aluminum
4. cimetidine
5. esomeprazole
6. saliva substitute
7. magaldrate
8. sodium bicarbonate
9. famotidine
10. misoprostol

Chapter 58: Laxatives and Antidiarrheal Agents

PATIENT TEACHING CHECKLIST

LAXATIVES

A laxative works to prevent constipation and to help keep the gastrointestinal (GI) tract functioning on a regular basis. It is used when straining can be dangerous or when a situation arises that constipation might occur.

Common effects of this drug include:

- Diarrhea—Have ready access to bathroom facilities. Consult with your health care provider if this becomes a problem.
- Dizziness, weakness—Change positions slowly; if you feel drowsy, avoid driving or dangerous activities and driving.

Report any of the following to your health care provider: sweating, flushing, dizziness, muscle cramps, excessive thirst.

Increase your intake of dietary fiber and fluid; try to maintain daily exercise to encourage bowel regularity.

Tell any doctor, nurse, or other health care provider that you are taking this drug.

Keep this drug, and all medications, out of the reach of children.

Special information regarding your situation:

- Take the capsule at bedtime and allow yourself time in the morning for it to work.
- Do not strain or push. If this dose does not work and you are still constipated or feel the need to strain, call the office.

WORD SCRAMBLE

1. cascara
2. loperamide
3. cisapride
4. psyllium
5. senna
6. metoclopramide
7. opium
8. docusate

TRUE OR FALSE

1. F   2. T   3. T   4. F   5. T   6. F   7. F   8. T

CROSSWORD PUZZLE

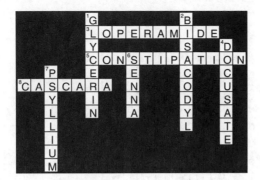

Chapter 59: Emetic and Antiemetic Agents

LISTING

1. Ingestion of caustic or corrosive mineral acid
2. Ingestion of a volatile petroleum distillate
3. Comatose or semicomatose patient
4. Signs of convulsions

CROSSWORD PUZZLE

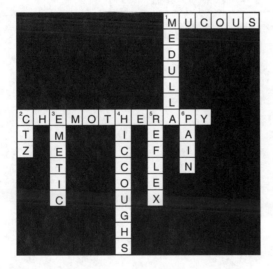

FILL IN THE BLANKS

1. vomiting
2. Ipecac syrup
3. Antiemetics
4. vomiting reflex
5. CTZ, medulla
6. pain, chemicals, uterine stretch
7. CNS depression
8. Photosensitivity

WORD SEARCH

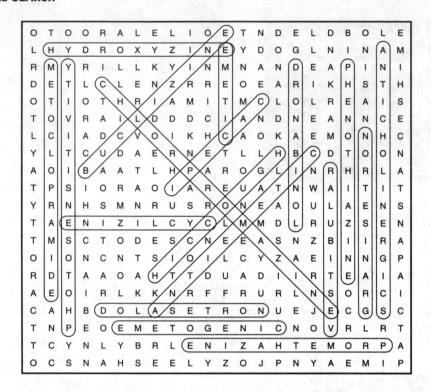